Social Work, Health and Equality

Deepening health inequalities, the restructuring of the welfare state involving the fragmentation of social work as a recognisable discipline and popular disaffection with health and welfare professionals underline the need to rethink social work's contribution to people's health.

In three main ways *Social Work, Health and Inequality* suggests what social work can contribute to people's health:

- the magnitude of the profound and unjust human suffering which arises from the impact of social inequalities on health should be a matter of urgent concern to social workers.
- through focusing on this problem, social work can make a significant contribution to more equal chances and experiences of health and illness.
- to make such an impact requires major shifts in the conceptualisation, practice and organisation of social work.

Social Work, Health and Equality will be essential reading to trainees and professionals in social work and health care.

Eileen McLeod is Senior Lecturer in the Department of Applied Social Studies, University of Warwick and **Paul Bywaters** is Head of Social Work, Coventry University.

The State of Welfare
Edited by Mary Langan

Throughout the Western world, welfare states are in transition. Changing social, economic and political circumstances have rendered obsolete the systems that emerged in the 1940s out of the experiences of depression, war and social conflict. New structures of welfare are now taking shape in response to the conditions of today: globalisation and individuation, the demise of traditional allegiances and institutions, the rise of new forms of identity and solidarity.

In Britain, the New Labour government has linked the projects of implementing a new welfare settlement and forging a new moral purpose in society. Enforcing 'welfare to work' on the one hand, and tackling 'social exclusion' on the other, the government aims to rebalance the rights and duties of citizens and redefine the concept of equality.

The State of Welfare series provides a forum for the debate about the new shape of welfare into the millennium.

Titles of related interest also in *The State of Welfare* series:

Taking Child Abuse Seriously
The violence against children study group

Women, Oppression and Social Work
Edited by Mary Langan and Lesley Day

Managing Poverty: The Limits of Social Assistance
Carol Walker

Towards a Post-Fordist Welfare State?
Roger Burrows and Brian Loader

Working with Men: Feminism and Social Work
Edited by Kate Cavanagh and Viviene E. Cree

Social Theory, Social Change and Social Work
Edited by Nigel Parton

Working for Equality in Health
Edited by Paul Bywaters and Eileen McLeod

Social Action for Children and Families
Edited by Crescy Cannan and Chris Warren

Child Protection and Family Support
Nigel Parton

Social Work and Child Abuse
David Merrick

Towards a Classless Society?
Edited by Helen Jones

Poverty, Welfare and the Disciplinary State
Chris Jones and Tony Novak

Welfare, Exclusion and Political Agency
Edited by Janet Batsleer and Beth Humphries

Social Work, Health and Equality
Eileen McLeod and Paul Bywaters

Social Work, Health and Equality

Eileen McLeod and Paul Bywaters

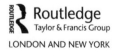
Routledge
Taylor & Francis Group

LONDON AND NEW YORK

First published 2000 by Routledge
2 Park Square, Milton Park, Abingdon, Oxon OX14 4RN

Simultaneously published in the USA and Canada
by Routledge
711 Third Avenue, New York, NY 10017

*Routledge is an imprint of the Taylor & Francis Group,
an informa business*

© 2000 Eileen McLeod and Paul Bywaters

Typeset in Times by Bookcraft Ltd, Stroud

British Library Cataloguing in Publication Data

A catalogue record for this book is available from the
British Library

Library of Congress Cataloging in Publication Data

A catalog record for this title has been requested

ISBN 0-415-16489-3 (hbk)
ISBN 0-415-16490-7 (pbk)

To Anna McLeod and Bruce and Margaret Bywaters

Contents

Tables

The state of welfare
Series editor's preface

State welfare policies reflect changing perceptions of key sources of social instability. In the first half of the twentieth century – from Bismarck to Beveridge – the welfare state emerged as a set of policies and institutions which were, in the main, a response to the 'problem of labour', the threat of class conflict. The major objective was to contain and integrate the labour movement. In the post-war decades, as this threat receded, the welfare state became consolidated as a major employer and provider of a wide range of services and benefits to every section of society. Indeed it increasingly became the focus of blame for economic decline and was condemned for its inefficiency and ineffectiveness.

Since the end of the Cold War, the major fear of capitalist societies is no longer class conflict, but the socially disintegrative consequences of the system itself. Increasing fears and anxieties about social instability – including unemployment and homelessness, delinquency, drug abuse and crime, divorce, single parenthood and child abuse – reflect deep-seated apprehensions about the future of modern society.

The role of state social policy in the Clinton–Blair era is to restrain and regulate the destructive effects of market forces, symbolised by the Reagan–Thatcher years. On both sides of the Atlantic, governments have rejected the old polarities of left and right, the goals of both comprehensive state intervention and rampant free-market individualism. In its pursuit of a 'third way' the New Labour government, which came to power in Britain in May 1997, has sought to define a new role for government at a time when politics has largely retreated from its traditional concerns about the nature and direction of society.

What are the values of the 'third way'? According to Tony Blair, the people of middle England 'distrust heavy ideology', but want 'security and stability'; they 'want to refashion the bonds of community life' and, 'although they believe in the market economy, they do not believe that the only values that matter are those of the market place' (*The Times*, 25 July 1998). The values of the 'third way' reflect and shape a traditional and conservative response to the dynamic and unpredictable world of the late 1990s.

The view expressed by Michael Jacobs, a leading participant in the revived Fabian Society, that 'we live in a strongly individualised society which is falling apart' is widely shared (*The Third Way*, Fabian Society). For Jacobs, the fundamental principle of the 'third way' is 'to balance the autonomous demands of the individual with the need for social cohesion or "community"'. A key New Labour concept that follows from this preoccupation with community is that of 'social exclusion'. Proclaimed the government's 'most important innovation' when it was announced in August 1997, the 'social exclusion unit' is at the heart of New Labour's flagship social policy initiative: the 'welfare to work' programme. The preoccupation with 'social exclusion' indicates a concern about tendencies towards fragmentation in society and a self-conscious commitment to policies which seek to integrate atomised individuals and thus to enhance social cohesion.

The popularity of the concept of social exclusion reflects a striking tendency to aggregate diverse issues so as to imply a common origin. The concept of social exclusion legitimises the moralising dynamic of New Labour. Initiatives such as 'welfare to work', targeting the young unemployed and single mothers, emphasise individual responsibility. Duties – to work, to save, to adopt a healthy lifestyle, to do homework, to 'parent' in the approved manner – are the common themes of New Labour social policy; obligations take precedence over rights.

Though the concept of social exclusion targets a smaller section of society than earlier categories such as 'the poor' or 'the underclass', it does so in a way which does imply a societal responsibility for the problems of fragmentation, as well as indicating a concern to draw people back – from truancy, sleeping rough, delinquency and drugs, etc. – into the mainstream of society. Yet New Labour's sympathy for the excluded only extends as far as the provision of voluntary work and training schemes, parenting classes and drug rehabilitation programmes. The socially excluded are no longer allowed to be the passive recipients of benefits; they are obliged to participate in their moral reintegration. Those who refuse to subject themselves to these apparently benign forms of regulation may soon find themselves the target of more coercive interventions.

There is a further dimension to the 'third way'. The very novelty of New Labour initiatives necessitates the appointment of new personnel and the creation of new institutions to overcome the inertia of the established structures of central and local government. To emphasise the importance of its drugs policy, the government has created the new office of Drugs Commissioner or 'Tsar', and prefers to implement the policy through a plethora of voluntary organisations rather than through traditional channels. Health action zones, education action zones and employment action zones are the chosen vehicles for policy innovation in their respective areas. At higher levels of government, semi-detached special policy units, think-tanks and quangos play an increasingly important role.

The *State of Welfare* series aims to provide a critical assessment of social policy in the new millennium. We will consider the new and emerging 'third way' welfare policies and practices and how these are shaped by wider social and economic changes. Globalisation, the emergence of post-industrial society, the transformation of work, demographic shifts and changes in gender roles and family structures all have major consequences for patterns of welfare provision.

Social policy will also be affected by social movements – the demands of women, minority ethnic groups, disabled people, as well as groups concerned with sexuality or the environment. *The State of Welfare* series will examine these influences when analysing welfare practices in the first decade of the new millennium.

Mary Langan
February 1999

Acknowledgements

We would like to thank many people for the help they have given in the preparation of this book, not least Mary Langan, the series editor, who has supported us from the start. Our respective employers, the University of Warwick and Coventry University, have given us encouragement and tangible assistance in the form of study leave. Library staff, particularly in Inter-library Loans and Official Publications and Statistics at Warwick, have been unfailingly efficient and friendly. Sonia Higgins word-processed for us throughout, speedily, skilfully and with consistent good humour; we owe her a particular debt.

Our colleagues have also provided significant support. Audrey Mullender, Helen Roebuck, Phillip Scullion and Denise Tanner offered their expertise at critical moments. Several people have provided valuable help as research assistants: Chantal Austin, Ravinder Atwal, Robert Gunn and, especially, Corinne Wilson. Others read and commented on drafts of the text: Meg Bond, Ben Grey, John Harris, Lesley Pehl and Alison Powell. This was done firmly but with encouragement, sometimes in immense detail and at very short notice; we are very grateful to them. We would also like to thank all the students who have helped to shape our ideas through discussion in teaching sessions on health and social work.

We have both been generously and robustly sustained at home, in particular by Anna McLeod and Olwen Haslam. Although we have reversed the usual alphabetical order of our names as authors, the work and the responsibility belongs equally to both of us.

Chapter 1

Inequalities in health

A social work issue

INTRODUCTION

Physical health is a site of social inequality. Unequal social relations create unequal chances of staying alive, unequal possibilities of health across lifetimes and inequalities in the experience of ill health. Profound, unjust suffering results. Social work in its own right can contribute to changing this situation: to creating greater equality in physical health. Yet this dimension to practice has barely gained recognition within social work, despite its crucial importance for people's well-being. In this book we examine the devastating impact of social inequalities on physical health, how social work generally – not simply in health care settings – may tackle this, and how such practice can be developed.

We focus specifically on health inequalities as a key issue for social work, for three fundamental reasons:

- The unjust, unnecessary suffering resulting from socially-constructed inequalities in physical health should be a cause of concern to social workers.
- Social work is implicated in processes which produce and maintain such inequalities.
- Social work can make its contribution to a more equal experience of physical health.

We now introduce each of these main themes in turn.

HEALTH INEQUALITIES: A CAUSE FOR CONCERN

A major social problem

Reducing health inequalities, primarily through addressing social inequalities, became central to the rhetoric of health policy following the advent of the Labour administration in 1997 (Department of Health (DoH) 1997a and 1998a).[1] Moreover social work, through independent sector and statutory social services, was seen to have a key role to play in this, with local authority departments being given joint lead responsibility with the NHS for meeting health inequality targets (DoH 1998b). However, these developments should not be read as representing a thoroughgoing, explicit and informed engagement on the part of social work with tackling social inequalities to promote greater equality in physical health. In social work discourse in the UK, attention to physical health – never mind the consequences of practice for health inequalities – remains marginal, as it has been over the past thirty years (Bywaters 1986 and 1996; McLeod and Bywaters forthcoming). Moreover, social work's general concern with different dimensions of oppressive social relations has not resulted in consideration of inequalities in physical health. Yet this constitutes a major social problem, characterised by widespread, pervasive suffering.

In Chapter 2 we detail how socially created and socially constructed inequalities in health have a profound impact on people's lives. At its most stark, social conditions affect how long people live. Nor are differences in life expectancy a matter of a few weeks or months. In 1991–3, men aged 20 in Social Class I had a life expectancy five years longer than men in Social Class V (Smith 1996). 'People may appreciate what a five-year gap in life expectancy means by understanding that if we were to cure cancer then life expectancy in Britain would go up by only about three years' (Macara, quoted in Smith 1996: 9).

These pronounced differences in life chances in the UK according to people's socio-economic position are found throughout the age range. A child's chances of dying in the first year of life are twice as great in Social Class V as in Social Class I. Children in Class V are almost five times as likely as a child in Class I to die from being hit by a car, over eight times as likely to die from a fire, over twice as likely to die from a respiratory condition (Roberts and Power 1996).

Not only is life expectancy linked to social circumstances but there are also extensive inequalities in people's chances of experiencing serious illness. Steep class-gradients are apparent across most major long-term and life-threatening illnesses, including heart disease, stroke, respiratory disease and lung cancer, with widespread and devastating effects on people's lives.

> For example, in 1996 among the 45 to 64 age group, 17 per cent of professional men reported a long-standing limiting illness compared to 48 per cent of unskilled men. Among women, 25 per cent of professional women and 45 per cent of unskilled women reported such a condition.
>
> (Independent inquiry (The Acheson Report) 1998: 14)

Multiple dimensions of social inequality and discrimination crosscut health. These result not only in unequal chances of maintaining good health but also in inequalities in accessing treatment, in securing the resources necessary to recovery or to a good quality of life in cases of serious illness, and in receiving high-quality care in terminal illness (Arber and Ginn 1991; Graham 1993; Grande *et al.* 1998; Marmot and Shipley 1996; Nazroo 1997). For example, the Acheson Report (1998: 99) concludes that:

> people from minority ethnic groups are more likely ... to: find physical access to their general practitioner (GP) difficult; have longer waiting times in the surgery; feel that the time spent with them was inadequate; and be less satisfied with the outcome of the consultation.

We can become immune to such findings, but they are evidence of lives cut short, or lived with unnecessary suffering and struggle.

Lay health work against powerful odds

The complex and intimate consequences of social inequalities for physical well-being are further revealed in the way they permeate 'lay health work'. (Stacey 1988). While the contribution of health and social care professionals is significant, the bulk of the work of maintaining health and managing illness, as we will show throughout, is done by lay health workers – lay people working on a day-to-day basis for their own or other people's health. For example, as Graham's

(1993) work has revealed, mothers parenting in poverty are constantly making hard choices about how they will meet their children's needs for the food, shelter and care which are fundamental to their health. Such choices, when constrained by inadequate material resources, may paradoxically draw the women concerned into apparently 'unhealthy' behaviours:

> 'I buy half a pound of stewing meat or something and give that to Sid and the kiddies and then I just have the gravy – before I used to buy soya things and substitutes to meat but I can't afford that now.'
>
> (Graham 1993: 160)

> 'When they are all screaming and fighting in here and in the kitchen, I'm ready to blow up so I just light up a cigarette. It calms me down when I'm under so much stress.'
>
> (Graham, 1993: 182)

As reflected here, in grappling day in, day out with the damaging effects on health of social inequalities, lay health workers are engaging with powerful social forces. The first of these is the economic system as a whole, which impacts directly on health chances through the unequal distribution of income and wealth, as well as through inequitable opportunities for work and job security. The second is the 'health industry', which feeds into and compounds socially created inequalities in health. The large and growing commercial health market, for example, exploits the notion of individualised responsibility for health through the promotion, at a premium, of 'healthy food', over-the-counter medication, the 'fitness/beauty' industry and private health care. This 'commodification' of health, as Crawford (1980) has described it, creating the expectation that health can (and should) be purchased, has a powerful ideological function as well as reinforcing inequalities in health according to the ability to pay.

A third social force with adverse consequences for equalising health chances, put simply, combines two functions identified as being fulfilled by the state in the context of capitalism. These are to foster 'accumulation and legitimation'.

> Under the first function, the state has to maintain and promote those social and economic circumstances in which profitable private capital accumulation can take place. However, under the function of

legitimation, the state must attempt to preserve and promote the general conditions of social harmony.

(Turner 1995: 179)

The significance of these roles was exemplified in the performance of the Conservative government in the UK across the 1980s and 1990s. Policies favouring the 'accumulation' agenda resulted in widening inequalities in the distribution of material and social resources (see Chapter 2). Accumulation was enhanced by government measures to – for example – control public expenditure, such as the detachment of state pension increases from average earnings; keep down wage levels, through sanctioning high rates of unemployment; transfer responsibility from the NHS to means-tested social services and to informal care; and promote private health and social care (Bywaters and McLeod 1996a). These developments were associated with a consequent widening in health chances between advantaged and disadvantaged sections of society (Wilkinson 1996a). Yet while instrumental in tilting the odds against physical well-being for large sections of the population, the government's discourse was characterised by a diversionary emphasis on health as a matter of personal responsibility or irresponsibility (DoH 1992) and by the use of health 'variations' as the officially preferred term to neutralise evidence of structurally created inequalities (DoH 1995a).

SOCIAL WORK: COMPOUNDING HEALTH INEQUALITIES

Inequality in physical health requires attention from social workers because of the gravity of the damage it inflicts on people's welfare and because of its socially constructed nature. It also demands attention because social work is itself implicated in the processes which produce and maintain such inequalities. We analyse this tendency in detail in Chapters 3 to 6. Here we indicate the extent to which it is institutionalised in practice.

A neglected issue at the heart of practice

Professional social work has shown a lack of awareness of the issue of inequalities in physical health despite the significance of this issue in the lives of the vast majority of its own service users, in whose experience the unequal social conditions which have such threatening and damaging effects on health are almost universal. Although there is relatively little systematic analysis of contact with social workers by social status (partly because most service users exemplify those groups not well recognised in statistics based on the employment of the male head of the household: Graham 1995) there is evidence of extensive poverty and deprivation. For example, studies in Strathclyde in the 1980s found that around 80 per cent of all service users were living on social security benefits and most on means-tested benefits (Becker 1997). Most children enter the care system from a family living in poverty (Bebbington and Miles 1989), while families with disabled children are disproportionately likely not to have the material resources to be able to sustain a healthy standard of living (Joseph Rowntree *Findings* 1998a).

Moreover, the few studies which analyse the health of service users show that the majority are either currently living with illness or caring for someone in poor health, often jeopardising their own health in the process. Corney's (1985) analysis of referrals to a generic intake team found that less than 10 per cent were free from physical symptoms, while almost two-thirds described themselves as suffering from a profound health problem. Redmond *et al.* (1996) investigated untreated health problems in seventy-seven older people receiving home care. Sixty-eight were assessed as likely to benefit from further intervention. In total 192 referrals were made. Studies of the outcome of caring for someone with a long-term illness in the absence of adequate material and personal support consistently demonstrate adverse consequences for carers' health (Anderson and Bury 1988; Spackman 1991).

A problematic record

Although the negative association between social inequalities and health is manifest in the lives of users of its own services, social work's record of addressing such situations is problematic. This is epitomised in the following two issues. First, social work has failed to implement measures to combat poverty as a consistent and central feature of practice (Becker 1997; Davis and Wainwright 1996), while too often adopting a pathologising, individualistic approach (Jones 1997). In Clark and Davis' (1997) survey of social workers' approaches to poverty, a depressing picture of the absence of even preliminary engagement with this issue was found. Limited awareness of poverty as a social problem and its significance in the daily lives of service users was accompanied by underestimation of levels of debt. Attempts to maximise income were far from routine – not surprising when almost half the employers questioned did not regard addressing relative poverty as an appropriate role for social workers.

Second, social work's record has also proved questionable in ensuring equality in access to, and in the experience of, the community-based domiciliary day-care and residential services which provide much-needed sources of practical, emotional and social support for people living with ill health. To give one example, successive studies have shown differential levels of information about services between minority ethnic groups and the majority population, and amongst minority groups in general. Coupled with institutionalised barriers to access this has resulted in inequalities in the use of mainstream services, not adequately compensated for by a 'special projects' approach which has often been dependent on temporary and vulnerable funding arrangements (Butt and Mirza 1996).

A bad situation exacerbated

Moreover, through the role assigned to it by state policies social work has been sucked into exacerbating social inequalities, with adverse consequences for health. As highlighted earlier, through the 1980s and 1990s state policies in Britain intensified social and economic inequalities. This process was also marked by a developing programme designed to individualise, domesticate, privatise and commercialise health and welfare provision, resulting in a worsening experience of ill health for the least powerful members of society. Social workers were drawn into this process of restructuring the state's role in welfare provision. This led to such trends in local authority social work as: gatekeeping increasingly inadequate financial resources; targeting at the expense of prevention; and a narrowed repertoire of intervention reflecting a more bureaucratised approach (Lymbery 1998; Means and Smith 1998; Parton 1996).

Despite identifying social work as necessary to its programme for tackling health inequalities, current welfare policy is characterised by some significant continuities with that of the previous administration. There remains a strong emphasis on individual, family and community responsibility; a focus on containing risk and dangerousness; and an expectation that social workers will act as managers of rationed provision with narrow eligibility criteria. Within this conception social work continues to occupy an 'essentially contested and ambiguous position ... between the respectable and the dangerous classes' (Parton 1996: 6); a balancing act characterised as protecting the vulnerable, while not undermining the independence of the private citizen in providing for their own and their family's welfare. This approach is manifest in the government white paper 'Modernising Social Services' (DoH 1998c) and linked policy documents which emphasise the management and regulation of social care provision rather than a substantial redistribution of material and social resources to underwrite service users' welfare.

SOCIAL WORK: CONTRIBUTING TO GREATER EQUALITY IN HEALTH

A positive contribution

Uncovering social work's complicity in perpetuating inequalities in physical health is a necessary prerequisite for establishing how social work in its own right can make a positive impact. In Chapters 3 to 6 we set out social work's positive contribution to greater equality in physical health. This is evident across four key dimensions: health creation and maintenance (Chapter 3); the experience of illness at home (Chapter 4); ill health in hospital (Chapter 5); and facing life-threatening illness (Chapter 6). In exploring each of these dimensions we:

- examine the conditions under which lay health work is carried out;
- discuss internal and external obstacles to social work intervention; and
- analyse examples of, and possibilities for, social work practice contributing to greater equality in health.

We demonstrate that only if social work redresses social disadvantage and explicitly tackles health inequalities can it play a significant role in producing more equal chances of physical health and greater equity when ill.

Characteristic elements of the type of practice which brings this about are:

- a direct contribution to increasing the material, environmental, personal and social resources required: for example, maximising income, securing safe appropriate accommodation, strengthening interpersonal and social support and improving access to information;
- collaboration in building up the infrastructure of interest groups, locality-based activism or self-help organisations in the interests of redressing discrimination; and
- advocacy and brokerage with the professionals concerned to ensure greater equity in accessing available professional care and treatment and in the quality of care received.

We do not focus on the social construction of mental health, which has already been the subject of considerable attention in social work. However, in addressing inequalities in physical health we are not endorsing a false mind–body dichotomy (Bendelow 1998). This reflects our view that the boundaries between physical health and the experience of emotional well-being are permeable. Our discussion testifies to the extent to which physical and emotional experiences interact as conduits of the adverse effects of oppressive social relations.

Social work 're-formed'

Notwithstanding the limitations outlined earlier, the current policy context is more favourable for social work's contribution to the objective of reducing inequalities in health than under the previous administration. First, as we have already mentioned, the current government is on record as giving high priority to tackling the impact of social inequalities on health as a central plank of health (and social services) policy (DoH 1997a, 1998a and 1998b). This recognition has been underlined by a number of connected policy statements and initiatives. Health inequalities are a focus for Health Action Zones (HAZs) (DoH 1997a), Health Improvement Programmes (HImPs) (NHS Executive 1998) and Primary Care Groups (PCGs) (DoH 1997a).

In addition, these initiatives involve a series of structural changes and operational imperatives which are designed to transform relationships between health and social services authorities. Symbolised by the *National Priorities Guidance* issued jointly to the NHS and social services (DoH 1998b), these include specific measures such as those requiring joint planning in a number of areas of policy, social services representation on PCGs, and the facility for pooled budgets.

However, our analysis of how anti-oppressive social work practice can target physical health necessitates new directions in practice, beyond the government's design. It also requires the definition of social work to be broadly drawn. Key features are as follows:

• Work aimed at securing a more equal distribution of the social and material resources which underpin health is found in local authority activity both within and outside social services departments. But it is also located in independent sector welfare agencies, in service user networks, self-help groups, community development projects and lay initiatives unaligned to formal social work agencies.

• Elements of practice not conventionally designated 'social work' in the UK are nevertheless integral to work which tackles socially constructed health inequalities. Such elements include renewed interest in collective self-help, information activism, non-violent direct action and rights work, and action research. Lay activism emerges as the driving force: refashioning the power relations, organisational forms, preoccupations, vocabulary and analysis of practice.

• Issues currently on the margins of social work also move to the centre: addressing poverty becomes of fundamental importance, as does countering the tendency to sideline anti-oppressive practice in order to conform with technocratic and managerialist objectives.

In alliance with disability rights

Social work action on inequalities in health is not antithetical to disability rights activism but complementary to it. Headway has been made in establishing that social work practice concerning physical or cognitive impairment and mental health should be predicated on an understanding of the social creation of inequality (see, for example, the work of Barnes and Shardlow 1996; Morris 1993; Oliver 1990). Our standpoint reveals how, in parallel to the relationship between disability and impairment, the experience of physical ill health is permeated by discrimination in interaction with disease. This is reflected in the socially created and unjust distribution of the incidence of physical illness, of physical suffering in ill health, and of death.

Work focusing on the social creation of inequalities in physical health complements the hard-won understandings gained by disability rights work. Our discussion opens up the fact that people's experiences of disability and of socially constructed illness have a simultaneous and compounding impact, and in doing so, extends analysis of the impact of unequal social relations to areas of experience currently acknowledged within the disability rights literature to be relatively untheorised (Barnes and Mercer 1996). Such areas include a focus on:

- the unjust, socially constructed distribution of disease which may lead to impairment;
- the social disadvantages that occur in the course of relatively short-term experiences such as acute illness (Dhooper 1990), childbirth (Oakley 1984) or surgical intervention (Henwood 1995);
- the actual experience of physical impairment, not just disablist responses to it, as bearing the imprint of social inequality (Pinder 1996). Crow (1996: 7), for example, argues for recognition that, through the suffering it represents, 'impairment in itself can be a negative, painful experience'. We would go further, and argue that impairment as a physical state is permeated by the impact of unequal social relations, quite apart from any disablist social responses. The likelihood of experiencing pain as a physical phenomenon (let alone its psychological dimensions), the intensity of pain and the length of time spent in pain in the course of illness are all mediated by the unequal nature of current social relations (see Chapter 6).

Action on inequalities in health is not represented by such a well-defined, broad, self-identifying social movement as is disability rights activism. However, as our discussion in subsequent chapters reflects, activists within contemporary movements for social equality, such as the women's movement, Black civil rights and gay, lesbian and bisexual rights, have identified physical health and illness as a site where social inequalities are embodied, amplified and need to be contested – as, for example, in the sexist, racist and homophobic disregard of treatment requirements (see, respectively, Doyal 1995; McNaught 1987; Watney 1996). Organising on health inequalities *per se* is also informed by analysis and practice honed by first-hand experience of oppressive institutional attitudes and practices and the action taken to combat them (See Positively Women 1994; Alcorn 1997). In parallel with disability rights activists, there is growing recognition among activists on health inequalities, that not only the social disadvantage associated with the onset or experience of ill health has to be tackled to end avoidable suffering, but also that equity in health should be identified as a civil right (Mann 1991).

SOCIAL WORK, HEALTH AND EQUALITY

The examples and evidence we examine constitute a case study based on the UK. However, the issues raised are of significance for the development of social work internationally. Across Chapters 3 to 6 our analysis shows that in its own right, social work, re-formed, can contribute to tackling inequalities in health and make a significant contribution to the well-being of the people concerned. The evidence we present makes the case that such a focus and activity should be integral to any social work practice concerned with promoting greater social equality.

Another issue to emerge is the powerful nature of existing constraints on effective action to tackle health inequalities, incorporating restrictions on the social work activities we describe. These include the continuing reluctance of the government of the day to embrace a thoroughgoing redistributive agenda; the power of the medical profession, in conjunction with the 'medical industrial complex', to dominate the discourse on health; the pervasive reach of a globalised capitalist economy; and the ideological dimensions of unequal social relations manifest in the exercise and experience of power dispersed throughout society.

We demonstrate that a further positive outcome of social work re-formed to address inequalities in physical health is that it is able to leave behind the exclusive and hierarchical forms of inter-professional practice that are currently its key health alliance, and create and enter into new working partnerships which will exert leverage on these daunting forces, on both a national and a transnational basis. So, for example, it can feed into international campaigns on environmental issues, to which social work in general is at present unaligned and unconnected. It can provide authoritative sources of first-hand evidence on the dire health consequences of inadequate income, and on discrimination by the medical and political establishment. It can facilitate the collective representation of local communities of interest at the level of policy-making and contribute to building and sustaining effective pressure politics. In Chapter 7 we provide case-study evidence of these processes in operation – a critical by-product of developing anti-oppressive practice on health.

The fundamental rethinking and redevelopment of social work's impact on physical health as a previously unrecognised aspect of anti-oppressive practice generates three major conclusions. First, the unjust human suffering which arises from the impact of social inequalities on health should be a matter of urgent concern to social workers. Second, through explicitly focusing on this problem and addressing social inequalities, social work can contribute in its own right to the creation of more equal chances and experience of health and illness. Third, in the process, social work can also engage with diverse, wider, egalitarian social movements to achieve greater equality in health.

Chapter 2

Inequalities in health

Oppression in bodily form

INTRODUCTION

In this chapter we underline the case that inequalities in health should be a central concern for social work. We give evidence of the extent of this major social problem and the complex ways in which health inequalities are linked with multiple dimensions of social inequality. We argue that oppression is physically embodied in the suffering involved in ill health and premature death. We present evidence of widening inequalities across the UK population and show how these inequalities are woven into the fabric of people's daily lives as they work to secure and maintain health for themselves and those close to them. We discuss the economic and policy backdrop to this daily labour of lay health work and argue that inequalities in health are not simply the visible outcome of a particular economic system but are part of the process through which the economic and political system is sustained. We focus on policy relating to health care as an example of the wider reconstruction of welfare.

This chapter prepares the ground for a detailed examination across Chapters 3 to 7 of the actual and potential role of social work in reducing health inequalities. It is not concerned with inequalities in the experience of illness, which are also the focus of later chapters, but primarily with inequalities in 'health chances': people's chances of staying well, getting ill or dying prematurely (Moore and Harrison 1995).

The production of health: Social, economic and environmental factors

In Britain, the Black Report on *Inequalities in Health* (Department of

Health and Social Security (DHSS) 1980) proved to be a landmark study, demonstrating that the NHS and social services had been ineffective in closing the gap in health between rich and poor (Davey Smith *et al.* 1990 and 1998a). Since then an extensive body of evidence on the association between social inequalities and inequalities in health has been developed (Whitehead 1987; Davey Smith *et al.* 1990; Smaje 1995; Watt 1996). In 1998 the government-commissioned review of research, the Acheson Report, concluded: 'The weight of scientific evidence supports a socio-economic explanation of health inequalities. This traces the roots of ill health to such determinants as income, education and employment as well as to the material environment and lifestyle' (Independent Inquiry 1998: xi).

The vast majority of the improvement in life expectancy in the UK over the last 200 years has resulted from changes in the material and environmental circumstances in which people live, with public health measures such as clean water, good sanitation, safe food and vaccination also playing a significant role (Gray 1993). Even within relatively prosperous, 'developed' economies with apparently comprehensive health care systems supported by 'scientific' medicine, health chances are tied to economic, social and environmental factors. These vital resources for human life are unequally distributed, not only in terms of social class but of other dimensions of social difference associated with 'race', gender, age, disability and sexual orientation. Patterns of health and illness in a population reflect the multi-layered impact of economic, political and cultural forms and practices. As Graham (1993) exemplifies, the combination of caring responsibilities, inadequate material resources and temporary accommodation constitutes a particularly powerful primary threat to health:

> 'I can't get registered with a doctor. I've lived here a year without one, and with a baby. He's been in hospital twice. He caught a virus from the hotel, which was growing in his bowel. He lost over six pound in a week. Then he had a blocked intestine so he was in hospital for nearly two weeks that time ... I feel so old, I mean I don't class myself as being young. I'm 34. But I don't know – I feel so old now, so very, very old.'
>
> (Miller 1990, quoted in Graham 1993: 175)

The primacy of economic, social and environmental factors is reflected in evidence that treatment-oriented health care has relatively little impact on the health chances of populations. In 1979

McKeown demonstrated that most of the reduction in morbidity and mortality due to infectious diseases such as TB and measles occurred before, rather than after, the introduction of effective drug treatments. More recent work on this issue has supported his view. As Mackenback *et al.* (1990) concluded, 'even among those conditions where the influence of medical care ought to be maximised, a review of studies shows that death rates are still more closely related to social and economic factors than to medical care variables' (quoted in Wilkinson 1996a: 66).

These arguments do not imply that medicine is of no benefit. They reflect a critical approach to equating the health of the population with the state of medical care or with the size or quality of the NHS. They look 'upstream' to the causes of inequalities in health, as well as 'downstream' to the lived experience of health and illness. As Wilkinson (1996a: 67) argues:

> The smallness of any influence which medical care may have on population health is not ... a reason for thinking it is ineffective. An army medical corps may do invaluable work on battle wounds and yet never be an important determinant of the number of casualties in a battle. In terms of civilian health, the battlefield is the social and economic circumstances in which we live.

It is the health consequences of deprivation, discrimination and inequality to which we now turn.

INEQUALITIES IN HEALTH CHANCES

Unequal health chances: Socio-economic factors

The dominant tradition in work on health inequalities in the UK has focused on links between social class and measures of mortality (death rates and life expectancy) and of morbidity (diagnosed illness). Criticisms of the validity of measures of social class based on male occupation have led to the examination of other measures of socio-economic status (Davey Smith *et al.* 1990 and 1998b). Paying attention to the non-employed – as the majority of social work service users are (Becker 1997) – reveals increased inequalities as well as the significance of dimensions other than occupation (Judge and

Benzeval 1993; Roberts *et al.* 1997). It is 'those occupying disadvantaged positions in the hierarchies of class, gender, "race" and disability who are over-represented among households on low income' (Graham 1995: 10).

Moreover there has been increasing recognition that 'medical' statistics of health and illness can illuminate only part of the picture (Graham 1993). This is reflected in evidence based on self-reported health status (such as General Household Survey data) and on qualitative data. We see all these sources as complementary.

However, whether relying on classification by occupation or by measures of deprivation, the evidence of substantial differences in mortality between those who are relatively well-off and those who are poor remains consistent across a range of data sources (Davey Smith *et al.* 1990; Drever and Whitehead 1997). For example, there is no main cause of death for which children in Social Classes IV and V have lower rates than those in Classes I and II (Woodrofe *et al.* 1993). The chance of a child from Social Class IV or V dying in the first year of life is over 40 per cent higher than for a child in Classes I and II (Independent Inquiry 1998). In the early 1980s, even before the rapid increase in childhood poverty which has taken place, death rates for children aged 1–15 in Social Class V were more than double those for Classes I and II, while death rates for adults classified as 'unoccupied', mostly economically inactive single mothers, who constituted 6 per cent of the population, were three times as great (Judge and Benezeval 1993).

Such inequalities exist throughout life (Arber and Ginn 1993) and are reflected in most of the major causes of death, including coronary heart disease, stroke, lung cancer, accidents, violence and suicide. There would have been over 17,000 fewer deaths per year from 1991 to 1993 in England and Wales if all men aged 20–64 had had the same death rates as those of Social Classes I and II (Independent Inquiry 1998). This translates into substantial differences in life expectancy: an average of five years more for men in Social Classes I and II, compared with those in Classes IV and V; a gap of three years for women (Drever and Whitehead 1997). Watt reports even greater differentials between districts. On average 'people in the most deprived areas of Glasgow die 10 years earlier than people in its affluent suburbs' (1996: 1026–7). Marmot and Shipley (1996: 1180) concluded that 'important socio-economic differences in mortality persist beyond retirement age ... On an absolute scale these differences increase with

age'. As Watt powerfully put it, 'dying before your time is the ulti-
mate social exclusion' (1996: 1027).

A similar picture of physically embodied social inequalities
emerges from diverse sources of evidence linking morbidity to social
class. Power *et al.* (1998), analysing data collected on over 17,000
children born in 1958, found that at ages 23 and 33, men and women
in Social Classes IV and V were twice as likely to report poor health.
At age 33 this accounted for more than one person in six in the
unskilled and semi-skilled groups. Moreover, many people who do
not report themselves to be in poor health are nevertheless living with
long-term illness (Bowling and Windsor 1997). Evidence of links
between illness and socio-economic status are paralleled in reports of
pain, tiredness, sleep disturbance and emotional distress; Davey
Smith *et al.* (1990: 374) concluded that 'the shorter lifespan in less
privileged groups seems to go with a longer period in poor health'.
The effects of occupational status and illness are circular. For example, manual workers are more likely than non-manual workers to be
forced out of work by chronic illness (Davey Smith *et al.* 1990). As
we discuss in Chapter 6, even when a diagnosis of terminal illness has
been given there are class-related differences in length of survival
(Cannon *et al.* 1994; Davey Smith *et al.* 1990).

In 'developed' countries, socio-economic inequalities affect rates
of ill health and death rates across society as a whole, not just among
those in relative poverty (Wilkinson 1996a). For example, the long-
term follow-up of a large cohort of civil servants by Marmot and colleagues found that each successive 'grade' of the service was linked to
better health outcomes than the one 'below' (Marmot *et al.* 1984;
Marmot and Shipley 1996). As the Independent Inquiry (1998: xi) put
it, 'these inequalities affect the whole of society and they can be identified at all stages of the life course from pregnancy to old age'.
Reducing health inequalities cannot be achieved just by targeting the
'socially excluded'.

Social class and deprivation do not only impact on health through
the effects of income differentials, but can also be seen to mediate the
impact of environmental conditions on health. There has been growing recognition of the negative effects on health, both current and
potential, of environmental pollution; for example, the impact of
global warming on the incidence of skin cancer, and of traffic pollution on respiratory disease (Friends of the Earth 1995). But evidence
is accumulating that lower socio-economic position can expose you
to greater risks. In Britain the concentration of cheaper, less well-

insulated inner-city housing stock close to higher traffic concentrations is implicated in the steep class gradient of the most severe form of asthma (Cochrane *et al.* 1994).

Moreover, the working and domestic environment contains health risks which reflect differentiated social position. Unskilled and other manual workers are particularly vulnerable to a range of pressures increasing the likelihood of workplace accidents. As Quick (1991: 87) shows, 'weaker unions, "speeding up" processes, more small firms, higher staff turnover, casual labour and contracting all have implications for safety'. At home, inadequate income increases the risk of the disconnection of water and fuel supplies, the 'voluntary' restriction of heating and washing or the use of heating and lighting methods which bring increased risks of fire (Ahmad and Walker 1997; Roberts 1997). As Graham (1993: 161) reports, parents, most commonly mothers, act to cut down bills while trying to minimise health costs: 'I put the central heating on for one hour before the kids go to bed and one hour before they get up. I sit in a sleeping-bag once they've gone to bed'; and 'When the children are in bed, I turn the heating off and use a blanket or an extra cardigan.' But such strategies are not always successful. The increased rate of death among older people in winter is partly attributed to hypothermia (Independent Inquiry 1998), linked to the combination of low income and a greater chance of living in accommodation which is difficult to heat.

Unequal health chances: 'Race'

A crucial development since the work of the Black Report has been the recognition that other dimensions to inequality, such as ethnic identity, affect people's health chances, cross-cutting and interlocking with the impact of social class and economic disadvantage. Again there are limitations in the methods of data collection which have been used.

The failure routinely to collect and analyse evidence about mortality and morbidity based on ethnic identity in the last three decades is not just disappointing; it reflects institutional racism (Graham 1995). Statistics collected by place of birth are of limited value in examining 'racial' differences in health in the UK when half the Black British population is UK-born (Fenton 1997). Nevertheless they provide evidence of excess mortality among men born in the Indian subcontinent and men and women born in Africa, Scotland and Ireland (Independent Inquiry 1998). Substantially raised rates of stillbirths and deaths in the first week of life are found when mothers have been born in the Indian sub-continent (Smaje 1995). Adult Punjabi Sikhs, Gujarati Hindus and Muslims from India and Pakistan have death rates from coronary heart disease around 40 per cent higher than the majority white population (NHS Centre for Reviews and Dissemination (CRD) 1996). People born in the Caribbean have twice the incidence of stroke compared to the general population (CRD 1996). Deaths associated with hypertension are four times higher in men and seven times higher in women (CRD 1996). Some groups also have substantially *lower* mortality rates from particular conditions than the majority population (for example, low rates of death from coronary heart disease amongst men born in the Caribbean), but this too has been the subject of little attention.

Analysis of data based on ethnic identity rather than on country of birth shows that members of African-Caribbean, African and Indian groups and, especially, those of Bangladeshi or Pakistani origin, have raised rates of limiting long-standing illness by comparison with the majority white population (Nazroo 1997). This reflects increasing evidence that the main reason why people from Black minority ethnic groups have unequal health chances is the association between 'race' and socio-economic status. Smaje (1995) and Modood *et al.* (1997) record the greater likelihood that people in Black minority ethnic groups will suffer material disadvantage as a result of discrimination than will their white British counterparts. Unemployment rates for most minority ethnic groups are considerably higher than for whites, and the gap grew during the 1980s. Differences are greater still amongst the young and long-term unemployed. When in work, disproportionate numbers of men from minority ethnic groups are in low-paid occupations, taking into account the level of their educational qualifications, and poor working conditions – shift work, night-work and homeworking – are more common. People from minority ethnic groups are more likely to have poor social security rights. Housing tenure also exhibits marked ethnic patterns, with the quality of housing in each sector tending to be poorer.

It is, therefore, not surprising that findings from Nazroo's (1997) comparative study of minority ethnic groups' health suggest that economic status is the key to differential chances of health – not only between members of minority ethnic groups and the majority population, but also between and within different minority ethnic groups. So, for example, people of Pakistani and Bangladeshi origin were found to be, on average, 50 per cent more likely to report ill health than the majority population, reflecting the evidence that over four-fifths of households in these communities have below half the average income (Modood *et al.* 1997). One of Ahmad and Walker's respondents described what the combination of poor health and poverty meant for her:

'It's a problem finding enough money to properly furnish my house, to help me. And finding enough money to go back to Bangladesh to see my other five children and getting my daughter wed. I need help to re-unite me with at least one of my sons so that he can look after me in my old age.' (Respondent, a Bangladeshi widow in her late 50s, with chest problems and severe money problems, whose sons have been refused entry to the UK.)

(Ahmad and Walker 1997: 151)

Indian and Chinese groups, whose income was closest to that of the majority population, were generally as healthy, while rates of heart disease amongst wealthy Pakistanis and Bangladeshis were little different from the majority population.

Self-assessed health shows similar substantial inequalities between the majority white population and minority groups (Rudat 1994), again largely attributable to the experience of people of Pakistani and Bangladeshi identity and, to a lesser extent, African-Caribbeans.

Unequal health chances: Gender

Gender inequalities in health chances are significant, but complex and insufficiently understood, with men having a substantially lower life expectancy – about five years (Independent Inquiry 1998) – but also higher rates of self-reported 'good' health from childhood onwards. Again the evidence needs careful reading. Differences can be relatively small. Arber and Ginn (1993) reported that for each five-year cohort in old age only about 5 per cent more women than men assessed their health as 'poor' or 'fair'. Bowling and Windsor (1997) interviewed almost 2,000 adults aged over 16 in 1996 and also found limited and variable gender differences in self-reported long-standing illness (Table 2:1). Of the illnesses mentioned, those involving the musculosekeletal system affected almost half those reporting ill health, with heart and circulatory, respiratory and digestive problems affecting between one in five and one in seven.

While levels of reported illness show little difference between men and women (see also Independent Inquiry 1998), there is evidence that women's health is more severely affected. By age 75 and over, the physical functioning of three-quarters of women, compared to half of men, was affected by their health status. There were statistical differences favouring men over 75 in the ability to climb stairs or walk half a mile, in role limitations attributable to physical health, in limitations in social functioning, and in pain and energy levels (Bowling and Windsor 1997).

Determining the extent of gender differences in health from both self-assessed and medically recorded data can be complicated by differences in the perceptions which men and women hold about their own health and in the way their health is perceived by doctors. Popay *et al.* (1993) found that the higher reporting of symptoms of affective disorders and minor physical morbidity by women compared to men reflected real differences in the number and severity of symptoms. At the same time her work has uncovered how women tend to ascribe profound and persistent fatigue to the unavoidable demands of motherhood, rationalising it as not a health problem and therefore not an appropriate issue for medical attention (Popay 1992). Gender bias is well evidenced in doctors' diagnostic processes and treatment decisions and in the drugs industry's investment in targeting medication on the basis of gendered stereotypes – for example, psychotropic drugs for women worn down by caring roles (Doyal 1995; Foster 1995).

Table 2.1 Reported long-standing illness by age and gender: percentage

Age	Gender	
---	Male	Female
16–24	19	25
25–44	29	27
45–54	44	48
55–64	52	54
65–74	64	56
75+	64	65

Source: Bowling and Windsor (1997)

Once again, gender differences affecting health chances are cross-cut by inequalities in socio-economic status, at home and at work. Women are more likely to live alone as lone parents or following the death of a partner in old age, to have caring responsibilities, which can mean that they put others health before their own, and to be living in poverty (Graham 1993). Graham details how women's financial and material circumstances are affected in multiple ways associated with women's traditional roles in the home and in providing care, with negative consequences for health. Women also experience relative disadvantage in work – lower wages, less security, worse terms and conditions, fewer career prospects, greater stress from juggling work with caring responsibilities – compounded by the inadequacies of the social security system on which they are more likely to be forced to depend, and by reduced access to credit.

> 'I find I get a lot of headaches and it's all down to stress. It's the situation I'm in … I mean it's the money and the situation that everything is my responsibility, you know. I never go out, never get time to relax … I think it's stress [that causes] headaches, high blood pressure, all this …'
> (Cohen *et al.* 1992, quoted in Graham 1993: 173)

Unequal health chances: Other dimensions

The Acheson Report focused on the influence of socio-economic factors on health inequalities, compounded by ethnicity and gender (Independent Inquiry 1998). While these are key aspects, other dimensions of socially structured inequalities which also impact on physical health are often ignored. For example, studies of people with mental health problems or learning difficulties rarely make links with physical morbidity or premature mortality (Littlechild 1996; Weich and Lewis 1998). Yet as Davis and Wainwright (1996) have shown, mental health service users face major difficulties in securing the basic resources necessary for good physical as well as mental health: sufficient food, adequate clothing, decent and affordable housing, employment, social and leisure activities. Other studies have also reported links between mental ill health and the factors which threaten physical health: low income, unemployment and financial strain (Weich and Lewis 1998). Moreover, particularly amongst older people (for example, Boneham *et al.* 1997), but also amongst homeless families (Cumella *et al.* 1998) and across the board (Corney

1983) people in contact with social work services commonly show evidence of poor physical and mental health. Yet physical morbidity and mortality amongst people with mental health problems is not a focus of attention, beyond concern about premature death from suicide (DoH 1992). Similarly the few studies of the physical health of people with learning difficulties show evidence of a substantial raised incidence of physical health problems, but these are not linked in discussion to wider issues of inequalities in mortality and morbidity (for example, Howells 1986; Rodgers 1994).

Difficulties in establishing differences in health chances linked to sexual orientation are also subject to the institutionalised discrimination of inadequate data collection. Graham (1995: 15) quotes the 1991 census report as having determined that 'cohabiting couples of the same sex were not recorded as such; instead, after clerical scrutiny of the forms, either the record of sex of one of the couple or the relationship was changed'. Nevertheless, the stresses resulting from officially sanctioned discrimination can be expected to have an impact on gay men's and lesbians' health; prospects in education and employment are liable to be negatively affected (Davies and Neal 1996) and there is evidence of raised rates of mental health problems, suicide and parasuicide amongst gay men, associated with homophobic behaviour, violence and fear of violence (Rivers 1995; Taylor and Roberston 1994).

The embodiment of oppression

Inequalities in material circumstances affecting, in combination, income, accommodation and the physical environment, act *directly* on health – through people's diet, through their capacity to keep warm, through dirty, insanitary and dangerous conditions. This is exemplified in comments reported by Kempson (1996: 41–3):

'It certainly affects your health … your body gets completely run down … you're not eating properly, you're not sleeping properly and you're not getting proper heat.'

'I'm on what you call a highline diet, with me diabetes. But some weeks it goes out of the window. You can't afford to buy a special diet for me … It is a very expensive diet. Sometimes I've had to really cut down with food … As a diabetic I shouldn't – I can't go without food. But the things I should really eat, I can't.'

'In bed it's freezing and if you saw the things I wear in bed to keep warm it's unbelievable. But I hurt when I'm not very warm, it's the arthritis. It really hurts when it's too blooming cold.'

'My asthma's been getting worse since I was homeless, my asthma's got worse and worse ... when I was on the street it was very bad.'

In addition, unequal economic and material circumstances impact *indirectly* on health chances through psychosocial pathways, 'through various forms of worry, stress, insecurity etc.' (Wilkinson 1996a: 184), again affecting life both at home and at work.

'We felt, you know, as if we were in the gutter. I've seen my wife sit in this chair with a piece of paper and pen working it out ... And that must have been a tremendous strain on her and she battled through. I'm sorry I can't do that. I'd much rather when it comes to a real push, go out there and jump under a bus ... when it gets to that stage I've gone to bed and ... unbeknownst to her ... I've prayed to God "Please let me have another [heart attack], let's get out of this".'

(Kempson 1996: 44)

Population studies have repeatedly found that psychosocial factors, such as low self-esteem, stressful 'life events', anger, lack of social support, low participation in community life, having little control over your work and insecurity, are all bad for health (Wilkinson 1996b).

'When they turned the water tap off, I felt very upset, I can't explain ... I feel very ashamed ... personally ashamed. I feel ashamed at myself. I couldn't manage to pay the water and the supply had been cut off.'

(Kempson 1996: 37)

'I have lost all my friends. I don't go out much now, but a few years ago when I used to go and see my friends, as soon as they saw me the first thing that struck them was maybe I was coming to borrow something. Even if I had come to say "Hello".'

(Kempson 1996: 30)

The health of civil servants who were told that they could anticipate job change and possible non-employment deteriorated by comparison with those remaining in stable employment before the material consequences of any job loss could take effect (Ferrie *et al.* 1995). Evidence from other studies of unemployment and job insecurity suggests that financial insecurity – in relation to the need for basic essentials as well as to the necessity of covering current commitments – is a health hazard (Bartley 1994).

> 'Every time you buy something, you count it up in your head just to make sure, when you get to the checkout, you've got enough … People like me – we do this every single day of our lives, the strain must tell somehow.'
>
> (Kempson 1996: 44)

The result is not only greater differentials in death rates but also increased stress and difficulties in everyday living: in young men 'rising suicide rates and increased crime, drug misuse and violence, in young mothers high levels of mental stress and anxiety which in turn may affect the development of young children' (Watt 1996: 1027).

> Little things that never mattered before are suddenly major issues and you fight over them. I fight with [my husband], I shout at the kids, he does as well and the kids cry. They probably don't argue any more than they used to, but because we're here all the time it seems like it.
>
> (Kempson 1996: 31)

In diverse ways, socially created inequalities are given physical expression, are embodied, in unequal health: in the length of people's lives and the physical and emotional quality – or suffering – experienced during life. As many social work service users could testify, 'Inequality may make people miserable long before it kills them' (Davey Smith 1996:988).

Moreover, health inequalities have been getting worse.

INCREASING INEQUALITIES

The impact of social inequalities on health has been graphically exemplified during the past two decades, with painful human consequences. For most of this period Britain's state policies, in concert with trends in other 'developed' countries (Mackenbach and Kunst 1997), deliberately increased social and economic inequalities

(Joseph Rowntree Foundation Income and Wealth Inquiry Group 1995b). The policies in question intensified a range of different dimensions to social disadvantage, through measures that – for instance – reduced the relative value of benefits for older and disabled people; tightened immigration policy; targeted particular social groups such as lone parents, gay men and lesbians; and tolerated higher levels of homelessness and unemployment (Bywaters and McLeod 1996a).

The most extensively documented evidence of growing inequality concerns increased inequalities in income, reflecting the New Right assumption that inequality stimulates economic performance (Glennerster and Midgeley 1991). For example, between 1983 and 1993 the incomes of the bottom 5 per cent of earners hardly changed, remaining at about £90 a week, while the incomes of the top 5 per cent rose nearly 50 per cent, to £550 per week. The number of people below the European Union (EU) poverty line increased substantially, with the proportion earning less than half the average income rising to 20 per cent of the population, compared with 6 per cent in the late 1970s (Johnson 1997). Meanwhile, the proportion of children being brought up in households dependent on income support tripled over a similar period (McKee 1993; Judge and Benzeval 1993), so that by the mid-1990s around one in three children was being brought up in a household with below half average income (Watt 1996).

The consequence of these deepening inequalities has been an intensification of the damage which unequal social conditions exact on health. Official data and research studies (summarised by Davey Smith 1996; Independent Inquiry 1998; Watt 1996; Wilkinson 1994a) have shown not only a rapid widening of health inequalities in the United Kingdom over the past twenty years but also, in some respects, increases in mortality amongst the most deprived sectors against a background of generally increasing life expectancy. Mortality rates in men in Social Class I fell by 36 per cent between 1970–2 and 1991–3, but increased by 2 per cent in Social Class V. The gap between Classes I and V widened from a twofold to a threefold differential (Smith 1996).

Cumulative insults

The evidence that widening socio-economic inequalities have produced widening health inequalities reinforces the arguments presented earlier, that social factors are the primary determinants of the health of a population. This evidence has also contributed to developing understanding of how social and economic conditions link with health outcomes. Davey Smith introduced the concept of 'cumulative socio-environmental insults' (1996: 987) to describe the processes involved.

For the major causes of death in the UK, such as heart disease, stroke, respiratory disease and some kinds of cancer, the influence of social factors – inequitably distributed – builds up over decades (Davey Smith *et al.* 1998c). The chances of contracting some illnesses, such as coronary heart disease and respiratory disease, have been shown to be related to experiences in both childhood and adult life. Others, such as stroke and stomach cancer, are linked to social circumstances in childhood but not significantly influenced by factors in adult life. In each of these cases the persistent influence of factors laid down in childhood means that overall mortality rates would not be expected to respond very rapidly to worsening social and economic conditions (Power and Matthews 1997; Power *et al.* 1996 and 1998). Moreover, it is hypothesised that the influence of important social assets such as education, welfare, the quality of housing stock and of the environment, together with biological assets, is 'not lost during periods of increasing social polarisation' (Davey Smith 1996: 987).The widening inequalities experienced during the past twenty years can be expected to take their toll in increased premature death from these conditions in the decades to come whatever subsequent policy initiatives are taken. This is partly why both the Black and the Acheson Reports emphasised improving the material conditions of mothers and young children as the crucial long-term measure (Davey Smith *et al.* 1998a). However, conditions mainly dependent on factors acting in adult life, such as violent deaths, including suicide, accidents and deaths from lung cancer, would be expected to be more rapidly 'responsive' to changing socio-economic policies (Davey Smith *et al.* 1998c).

These arguments are reflected in evidence about changes in the health gap over the past two decades, where the largest increases in inequality have come through mortality from accidents, violence and suicide (Watt 1996). Recent research into suicide and child deaths exemplifies this. Gunnell *et al.* (1995: 229) confirmed 'a strong relationship between suicide, parasuicide and economic deprivation in the 1990s' and suggested that the rise in suicide rates amongst young men (Beck *et al.* 1994) could be partly explained by the negative impact of social and economic policy changes which had resulted in increased homelessness, poverty and unemployment amongst this group.

Increased child and family poverty and homelessness have also had a rapid impact on child deaths. Overall, child deaths from injury and poisoning fell by 32 per cent in Social Class I and 37 per cent in Class II between 1981 and 1991, but by only 2 per cent in Class V (Roberts and Power 1996). Between 1979 and 1983 the difference in death rate between Classes I and V in deaths from injury in child-hood was three and a half times; by 1989–92 this had increased to five times. Moreover, in some respects childhood deaths amongst the poorest class actually rose: deaths from fires between 1981 and 1991 fell by 28 per cent in Social Class I, but rose by 39 per cent in Class V.

> Fire risk is greatest for those living in the poorest council accommo-dation and in temporary accommodation. The number of families de-clared homeless doubled between 1980 and 1991, with the number of households in temporary accommodation increasing nearly five-fold.
>
> (Roberts and Power 1996: 786)

This was undermining the government's own objective to cut the death rate from injuries in children aged under 15 by a third by 2005. Roberts and Power (1996: 784) concluded that this would 'be met for children in the non-manual social classes but not for those in the manual classes'. The significance for 'child protection' is that while something like two children a week die from 'child abuse', about thirty a week die in accidents (Woodrofe *et al.* 1993).

WORSENING INEQUALITIES: THE POLICY CONTEXT

The health chances of service users

The unnecessary suffering which health inequalities represents is the experience of nearly all those in contact with professional social workers, although systematic evidence of the health status and life expectancy of social work service users is scanty. First, the almost universal experience of poverty, briefly evidenced in Chapter 1, means that most service users' health is either threatened or already damaged. Second, most service users are also exposed to health damaging 'cumulative insults' because of other dimensions to inequality and discrimination interlocking with poverty, for example, as single parents, older people, members of Black and ethnic minority groups or because of mental ill health or learning disabilities. Third, poor physical health throughout the lifespan is often a key precipitating factor in social work contact, whether from inherited ill health at birth, the pressures associated with illness and injuries in childhood or the consequences of serious ill health in the absence of adequate social and material resources and health care provision in adult life and older age. The significance of ill health for social work service users has been reflected in legislation, from the 1948 National Assistance Act onwards, which has repeatedly placed duties on local authorities, and social services agencies in particular, to tackle different aspects of ill health.

The key threat to service users' health during the 1980s and 1990s has been the worsening and increasingly polarised economic conditions they have faced. However, under such circumstances, health and social services resources become increasingly significant in preventing the onset of, aiding recovery from and maximising quality of life with ill health. But here, too, the resources available to the majority of service users became increasingly scarce as the New Right developed its project of reconstructing welfare.

Reconstructing health and welfare

A key perception of the New Right was that welfare was not simply a set of social objectives to be paid for by the productive economy, but a central element in the economy as a whole and thus a significant lever of economic and political policy. Priority was given to the creation of the conditions under which it was believed economic growth could be maximised, including a healthy but compliant work-force, social control and stability, political legitimacy and high levels of demand – the conditions for accumulation and legitimation referred to in Chapter 1 (Hughes and Lewis 1998; Lewis 1998). The welfare state was presented as a powerful drag on economic growth, both directly, through demands on public expenditure which reduced individual freedom to spend, and indirectly, by creating a culture of dependency (Langan 1998).

Central to the strategy for breaking public expectations of the welfare state were three interlinked policy and ideological developments:

- curtailing increases in public expenditure on health and welfare;
- transferring welfare costs and responsibility from the public purse to private individuals; and
- the promotion of private provision in health and welfare services (Means and Smith 1998).

In each case change was relatively beneficial to those with comparatively high levels of income and wealth and disadvantaged those who were least well off. In the following discussion we examine the role of health policy in transforming expectations of the welfare state. The parallel example of social services is presented in Chapter 4.

Public expenditure: NHS underfunding

Since the mid-1970s successive administrations have emphasised the need to reduce – or curtail increases in – public expenditure on the welfare state in order to reduce personal taxation, particularly direct taxation (Langan 1998). The extent to which these objectives have been achieved is a matter for debate, but the equation was seen as essential to electoral success over this period and both the starting and higher rates of income tax saw substantial reductions.

However, although often represented politically as a 'bottomless pit', NHS expenditure in Britain has on the contrary been relatively modest over several decades. In 1996, UK public expenditure on health care was 6.9 per cent of gross domestic product (GDP) compared to the OECD average of 8.2 per cent, while the average spend in the 'Group of 7' economies was higher still at 9.4 per cent (BMA Health Policy and Economic Research Unit [BMA HPERU] 1998). Through the 1980s, in particular, public expenditure on health as a proportion of GDP was held almost constant against the long-term upward trend across almost all 'developed' economies.

In part this represents the relative efficiency of a comprehensive public health care system funded through taxation, including low administrative costs prior to the introduction of the internal market (Ranade 1998). But it also suggests persistent underfunding. NHS waiting lists as an indication of demand exceeding supply of treatment are controversial (Mohan 1995). Nevertheless, the 57,000 people who had been waiting over a year for NHS treatment in 1997 (*Guardian* 19 November 1997: 3) evidence a substantial gap between the desire for treatment and available resources. As Yates (1995) has shown, local inefficiencies in allocating services may account for part of the problem, but a major cause is shortage of resources, such as nursing or surgical staff or operating theatres, which reflects long-term and generalised underfunding.

Such waiting involves inequitable health risks and suffering. The College of Health's audit of sixty patients who had been waiting for hip or knee replacements for about a year found all had been experiencing pain, some to an overwhelming extent. 'I think of nothing but pain. It's ruining my life. My thoughts are just with pain' (Rigge 1994: 160). Several had routinely resorted to excessive dosages of powerful painkillers – very little NHS help with pain relief was evident. Many patients also experienced mobility problems and some were struggling to care for partners with even more severe physical impairment than their own. Nearly half lived alone and were experiencing considerable constraints on their ordinary routines.

Transferring responsibility: Domesticating health care

Chronic underfunding involves the transfer of costs and responsibilities from the NHS to private individuals. This transfer is partly enacted through the rapid reduction in lengths of stay in hospital and through increases in day-case and outpatient care, accompanied by the reduction in hospital beds seen over the past two decades (discussed in Chapter 5). Hospital beds were cut massively, from 7.1 per 1,000 in 1984 to 4.3 per 1,000 in 1994–5, while day cases doubled in the four years from 1990–1 to 1994–5(Ranade 1998). Although the reasons for these changes have been partially technological (and despite the reality that most people do not wish to stay in hospital any longer than is necessary), they have meant the discharge and home care of patients who are more ill than hitherto (Henwood *et al.* 1997). The rhetoric of technological advance, efficiency and patient choice has masked three key shifts of responsibility away from NHS provision: first, a shift of the demands and costs of care from the NHS to private individuals, to patients and informal carers; second, on occasion, a transfer to paid care in private nursing and residential homes or to paid (and voluntary) domiciliary care; and as such, third, the transfer of care from services free at the point of delivery by the NHS to care paid for wholly or partly by the patient and/or their family (Lewis and Glennerster 1996).

Privatising care

The provision of services which are not available when they are needed, to which entitlement is uncertain, which involve charges, contributions, top-up payments or complete financial responsibility – and which fail to adequately meet people's needs – generates circumstances in which private health and social care solutions are increasingly widely adopted. Lengthy waiting times for treatment are the major reason why people in the UK seek private treatment or purchase health insurance (Health Policy Network 1996). Meanwhile, in a vicious circle, the proportion of time which NHS consultants as a whole spend on private practice contributes to delays in NHS treatment (Yates 1995). Underfunding and the promotion of individualised rather than collective responsibility detaches from collective provision the interests of those who can afford to pay privately. It also weakens political support for universal provision, so that its defence can become a matter of sectional rather than national concern (Means and Smith 1998).

This situation is patently inequitable, in that more affluent sections of the population – including those whose employment carries private insurance – can circumvent delays and to some extent secure higher quality of care, by paying for private treatment. In 1980 only 6.4 per cent of the UK population had private medical insurance, but this had nearly doubled a decade later, by which time around a quarter of professionals, managers and employers were covered (Ranade 1998). Such a system disadvantages those who have less resources or in whom the commercial market has little interest: people who are chronically ill, who are poor, who are a 'bad risk', who live unstable lifestyles or in dangerous environments, who lack continuing employment or those alternative informal resources – including family and friends – on which so much health and well-being depends. 'It's frustrating when you want to get on with your life, but you can't afford thousands of pounds to have it done' (Rigge 1994: 162).

Health for sale

In a number of respects, therefore, how to fund health care and welfare in general can be seen as not so much a political problem for the New Right as an expression of its economic policy. In three ways, it can be seen that the approach taken supported private enterprise. First, the reconstruction of health care discussed above involved the direct transfer of provision to the profit-making sector. Second, the profits of the global health industry remained invisible and largely unquestioned. The expectation that 'developments' in medical technology meant that NHS inflation would be higher than general economic inflation was built into the government's calculations (Mohan 1995) almost without comment. There was little fundamental public debate about restricting or regulating medical 'advances' despite 'several recent cases of new technology ... which had been either highly cost-ineffective or where there was insufficient evidence about the likely benefits' (Pettinger 1998: 25). And third, the extension of private health care underpinned the creation of health as a commodity and the citizen as a health consumer. Not only were medical health care and commercial – over-the-counter – health products 'goods', to be purchased individually; 'health' itself became a medium through which the diet, leisure, beauty, fashion and media industries were promoted and extended.

> In the 1960s a list of 'health-related' commodities would have included items such as aspirins, TCP, Dettol and plasters. Today, however, it would include: food and drink; myriad health-promoting pills; private health; alternative medicine; exercise machines and videos; health insurance; membership of sport and health clubs; walking boots; running shoes; cosmetic surgery; shampoo (for 'healthy-looking hair'); sun oils; psycho-analysis; shell suits and so on.'
>
> (Burrows *et al.* 1995: 1–2)

Identity and status are marked not just by what we wear or what we can purchase, but directly through our bodies. Bodies become the malleable raw material of style, rather than the given skeleton on which fashion is overlaid. According to Glassner (1995), in America in the mid-1990s the fastest growing health creation industry was cosmetic surgery, already worth $5 billion a year, while the diet industry was more than double that size (Turner 1995).

This reflects the hidden ideological and financial power of the health industry as 'one of the most significant sectors of modern capitalism' (Rodberg and Stevenson 1977: 104). 'The power and size of the "medical–industrial" complex in the USA, for example, is now as great as that ascribed to the "military–industrial" complex in the 1960s' (Ranade 1998: 212), with health care alone involving some 14 per cent of total GDP. Even in a relatively 'socialised' health care system such as that of the UK, 52 per cent of NHS spending is calculated to involve purchases from the private sector (Salter 1995), while 17 per cent of total health expenditures are directly spent on private health care (Ranade 1998). Capitalist profit-making in the UK has taken the form of expanding the total market by promoting demand for new technologies and treatments (scanners, cosmetic treatments, Viagra, the new generation of anti-depressants such as Prozac), developing a private care market alongside the public health care system and penetrating the public care system (through, for example, the provision of drugs and technology, securing contracts for support services, agency staffing and direct care provision, and the private finance initiative) on a 'partnership' basis. Spending on health is not a drag on economic growth; on the contrary, it fuels it.

Cuts in public care provision remove a sense of social obligation and security in favour of an increasingly polarised, atomised and insecure society in which people are liable to see their priority as being to look after themselves and/or their immediate family. The 'disciplinary' consequences of this are clear, as the threat of losing work becomes a threat of losing insurance for future needs, losing access to care services; a threat to future quality of life. This reinforces the likelihood that workers will accept longer hours, reductions in sickness and other working conditions, the loss of trade union rights, less safe working practices and lower pay (Wainwright 1996).

A more socialist approach?

In some significant respects the incoming Labour administration in 1997 committed itself to reversing the trend towards increasing health inequalities.

- It highlighted the connection between relative poverty and health disadvantage (DoH 1997a), established a minister of public health to oversee research and policy initiatives to tackle this and set up the

Independent Inquiry into Inequalities in Health which reported late in 1998. A number of subsequent health policy initiatives, such as Health Action Zones (DoH 1997a), Health Improvement Programmes (NHS Executive 1998), Primary Care Groups (DoH 1997a), the green paper 'Our Healthier Nation' (DoH 1998a) and guidance on 'National Priorities' (DoH 1998b), reinforced this as a central strand of policy.

- It implemented a range of policies to tackle poverty, in particular:
    (1) the minimum wage;
    (2) the welfare-to-work (and child-care) programmes; and
    (3) the work of the social exclusion unit.
- After initially retaining the previous government's spending targets, it announced above-inflation increases in expenditure on the NHS averaging 4.7 per cent over the three years from 1999 to 2000, as part of the Comprehensive Spending Review (BMA HPERU 1998).
- It placed a high priority on reducing waiting lists.

However, substantial doubts remain as to whether this strategy constitutes a sufficient basis for substantial equalising of social and economic conditions. For example, as Hutton argues (*Marxism Today* 1998), why not target the overclass? Among criticisms of government policy are the following: first, while paid employment may constitute a significant site for tackling poverty, it cannot ameliorate the situation of those whose wage is inadequate for health, for whom work is not available, or who are outside the labour market because of age, poor health or incapacity. The government's programme to bear down on welfare spending includes measures aimed not only at promoting employment but also at restricting eligibility for benefits and uprating them. While accepting the public health minister's contention regarding entrenched inequality – 'To make a real difference we need long-term policies' (*Guardian* 9 September 1997: 3) – neither long- nor short-term measures to reduce relative poverty substantially by redistribution of income through the taxation system (Quick and Wilkinson 1991) have been mooted (*Guardian* 28 May 1997: 19 and 11 July 1997: 10). Indeed, redistribution has not been established as a policy or as an objective.

Second, the 5.8 per cent above inflation increase in NHS expenditure announced as part of the Comprehensive Spending Review for 1999–2000 represents £2.1 billion. An increase of over £7 billion (around 20 per cent) would be required for England alone to bring spending on health to the OECD average (calculations based on BMA

HPERU 1998). Again, at best, reversing decades of underfunding will be a long-term task.

Third, many of the other key elements of the previous administration's reconstruction of welfare, for example the privatisation and domestication of responsibility for health care, remain essentially unchallenged. Opportunities for making a profit from ill health, such as the private finance initiative established by the previous government, are promoted vigorously. This reflects a wider criticism of the government's approach, that it makes the twin assumptions that the interests of business and the poor can be held in common, while the essential nature of capitalism remains above consideration (Levitas 1996), and that globalised business is beyond the control of nation states (*Marxism Today* 1998). In 'Our Healthier Nation' (DoH 1998a) business is seen both as a beneficiary of preventive measures, through reduced sickness levels and NHS costs, and as a contributor to the public health, by looking after the health of employees and by offering skills of marketing and communication. This contrasts starkly with Townsend's (1995) prescription for investing in children's health through international economic action.

This will mean working with European allies to argue for:

- the introduction of forms of regulation of multi-national corporations;
- closing loopholes in cross-national taxation;
- protection of home-based companies and individual employees;
- using the Social Chapter to improve European labour law;
- promoting European trade union links;
- facilitating the internationalisation of democratic pressure groups;
- encouraging better relations between city authorities across countries; and
- fostering better First–Third world relationships.

(Townsend 1995: 11)

However, as we discuss in further detail in Chapter 7, since it remains uncertain whether the current administration's policies on equalising social conditions will prove to be minimalist or far-reaching, there is a case for social work contributing to sustaining pressure on the government to match its rhetoric with effective action.

CONCLUSION

The past two decades have confirmed the pervasive injustice of social, economic and environmental factors in the health of the population and of individuals. Government policies and ideologies designed to promote the interests of capitalist enterprise and economic growth have resulted in worsening social inequalities. These have not only brought about wider inequalities in health but, for some, have reduced life expectancy and increased morbidity. Amongst the casualties are actual and potential social work service users, commonly members of disadvantaged, marginalised and stigmatised populations who have been particularly affected by these changes. Moreover the reconstruction of welfare has further weakened the formal and informal resources and supports available.

As the preceding argument shows, policy on health and social care is not separate from, but a key element in, economic policy. Welfare is not above politics but a key site of ideological and political conflict. Health and social care are big business, wielding significant influence. The selling of health as a commodity, as something which can be purchased, marries with the individualising effects of underfunding public health and social care. Faced with inadequate collective provision, individuals will look after their own, feeding a private competitive market which, as it drives up expectations and creates 'need', will paradoxically also raise public health care costs (Turner 1995). In this twenty-first-century version of the survival of the fittest, it will be inadvisable to be poor and ill, but poverty and ill health will continue to go hand in hand.

Chapter 3

Health creation and maintenance

INTRODUCTION

A new direction for social work

After taking office, the Labour government signalled significant changes in policies aimed at creating and maintaining good health more equally in the population as a whole; changes with profound implications for social work. First, tackling health inequalities was moved to centre stage: one of the two declared aims of 'Our Healthier Nation' (DoH 1998a: 5) was to 'improve the health of the worst off in society and to narrow the health gap'. Second, the government argued that the primary means of reducing health inequalities was not through NHS policy and practice: 'Tackling inequalities generally is the best means of tackling health inequalities in particular. This means tackling inequality which stems from poverty, poor housing, pollution, low educational standards, joblessness and low pay' (DoH 1998a: 12). This agenda mirrored an international perspective on health creation in which health was seen as a collective good: in which one person's health should not be achieved either at the expense of others' ill health (equity) or at the expense of the environment (sustainability) (Dahlgren and Whitehead 1991; Labonte 1997).

These changes in policy direction have had two major consequences for social work. First, social work, in social services departments and the voluntary sector, is now expected to play a key role alongside others in developing strategies and implementing policies for maximising population health and reducing the 'health gap'. Second, any reductions achieved in social inequalities in general, in order to underpin this health-focused agenda, can be expected to bring benefits for social work service users.

However, of all the dimensions to social work's contribution to health which we discuss in this book, health creation remains the least visible in terms of mainstream practice. In recent years the perception has been that social work mainly becomes involved in health issues after illness has led to difficulties in daily living, rather than playing a primary role in preventing sickness and promoting good health. We argue that this view reflects a lack of awareness and analysis in social work itself of the interaction between lay efforts, inequitable material and social circumstances in the creation of good health, and that it fails to recognise the actual and potential impact of social work and social work organisations on health creation.

Leaving care: A threat to health

One brief example serves to underline the point. For most 16- and 17-year-olds, parents are still the main front-line health workers (Brannen *et al.* 1994). It is parents, mostly mothers, who are usually responsible for young people's diet, involved in negotiations about smoking and drinking and in detecting and advising about ill health, and who are active participants in arranging medical consultations. However, social work's record in 'parenting' young people who are leaving the care system does not compare well (Action on Aftercare Consortium 1996; Broad 1998). On two main grounds, practice can be identified as damaging to the health prospects of young people. First, care leavers have often been required to move out of their homes and live independently at an age much lower than 'loving parents' (DoH 1991a sec.1: 97) would expect. In 1996–7 records show that 3,400 young people left care at 16, while over 20 per cent of those leaving care over the age of 16 were already living 'independently' (McClusky and Abrahams 1998). Second, care leavers have commonly been discharged to exceptionally high levels of poverty, unemployment, homelessness or poor accommodation, early pregnancy or parenthood and social isolation (Action on Aftercare Consortium 1996; Save the Children 1995). For example, Broad (1998) found that around half of a large survey of care leavers were in temporary accommodation. These damaging social circumstances have been exacerbated by changes in public policy over the past twenty years which have reduced the employment opportunities and resources available to young people living independently (Broad 1998; Holtermann

1995). Thus care leavers have been expected to achieve independence despite the fact that damaging life experiences, reduced opportunities to acquire social and life skills and attenuated material and social support systems combine to render them more vulnerable than young people who have not been in the care system (Corlyon and McGuire 1997; DoH 1991b and 1991c).

These issues are rarely characterised in terms of the threats to health which they pose, but the well-being of young people who have been in care is clearly at risk. The stresses associated, not only with the reasons for initial entry to care but with what being in care entails – the multiple moves, lack of continuity in relationships, low educational attainment, reduced privacy, poor physical conditions and poverty levels of allowances for food, leisure, travel and holidays commonly experienced by these young people – are surely examples of cumulative environmental insults (Davey Smith 1996) and of the psychological intermediaries which link relative material deprivation with poor health outcomes (Blane *et al.* 1996; DoH 1991b and1991c). Moreover, social services' leaving care programmes have often barely begun to offer protection from the health-damaging material and social conditions commonly faced (Action on Aftercare Consortium 1996; Broad 1998) and, though care leavers are a focus of attention in the *National Priorities* (DoH 1998b) and *Quality Protects* (DoH 1998d) documents, targets set do not cover accommodation. The health consequences are manifold and dire. A consistent picture emerges of a high incidence of malnutrition, hypothermia, mental illness, sexual exploitation, susceptibility to physical attack, complications following drug use, serious consequences from otherwise minor infections and higher risk of HIV/AIDS, compounded by difficulties in accessing health care (Anderson *et al.* 1993; Boulton 1993; Centrepoint 1997; *The Big Issue in the North* 1997). These conditions also contribute to high death rates (Reuler 1993).

This example demonstrates both the relevance of social work to health creation and that social work can be involved in practice which has damaging rather than protective consequences. In doing so it also implies three key features of the social context in which social work contributes to health creation:

• the central role played by lay people (adults and children);
• the crucial significance of (unequally distributed) social, economic and environmental conditions in supporting or undermining lay health work; and

- the relevance of social, economic and environmental policies and institutions, including social work and social work organisations, for health creation.

In the remainder of this chapter we first highlight lay people's active engagement in creating and maintaining health against the background of unequal social conditions. Second, we discuss the limitations of health promotion policies which focus on individual behaviour and action. Third, we analyse in more detail the changes in policy signalled by the government. Fourth, through some key examples of positive initiatives being taken by local authorities corporately, by voluntary agencies and by self-help activists, we examine how social work can make a positive contribution to more equal chances of securing and maintaining good health.

LAY ENGAGEMENT WITH HEALTH CREATION AND MAINTENANCE

Against the odds

The Jakarta Declaration on 'Health Promotion into the Twenty-first Century' identified as prerequisites for good health, 'peace, shelter, education, social security, social relations, food, income, empowerment of women, a stable eco-system, sustainable resource use, social justice, respect for human rights and equity,' and concluded, 'Above all, poverty is the greatest threat to health' (World Health Organisation (WHO) 1997: 1). At the local, personal level these necessities are reflected in the daily struggle most social work service users face in order to secure and maintain the money, housing, gas, electricity and water supplies, food and clothing and social support which underpin health. For many this is a struggle against inequitable conditions in the context of factors in the local, national and international social, physical and economic environment which are clearly beyond their control.

Nevertheless, for most individuals, the work to obtain such necessities and maintain health begins with self-care and care given to and received from those close to them. Lay people act to secure the essentials for health and take the hour-by-hour decisions which produce accommodation, meals, heating, relationships, advice and information. This lay work goes on throughout life. Mayall's enquiries of primary school children showed that their understanding of the home as 'the principal site for health care and for learning health knowledge and behaviour' (1993: 482) was not just due to their parents' (mainly mothers') roles, but because these children perceived themselves as active workers for their own health. As one 9-year-old child said, 'We're keeping ourselves healthy by doing things ourselves. It's my body so it's my job' (Mayall 1993: 473). At the other end of the age range, the Health and Lifestyle survey reported in Sidell (1995) found that as many people over 65 claimed that they made positive attempts to keep themselves healthy as did those in younger age groups, with over 60 per cent of both men and women acting positively to maintain their health.

Graham's work (1984, 1987 and 1993) has highlighted this duality – individual action taken within the context of unequal social relations – as characteristic of lay engagement with health creation and maintenance: 'health-related behaviours are maintained within and against the constraining circumstances of everyday life' (Graham 1996: 176–7).

Informed choices?

Within the confines of inequitable social conditions, what appear to be health-damaging attitudes and behaviours can make grim sense. First, for example, the barriers to healthy behaviour may be excessive. The benefits of attendance at clinics or of buying and preparing 'healthy' food may be outweighed by the costs in time, energy and material resources, particularly for people without transport, with limited income and/or heavy caring responsibilities. In the case of young women in social services residential care, negotiating for contraception was fraught with obstacles linked to the actual or anticipated attitudes of care and health staff, while the unpleasant side-effects of contraceptive pills, injections or implants when finally obtained were often considerable (Corlyon and McGuire 1997).

Second, other goals may be more important than promoting health, or different health objectives may conflict. For the young women in care, the risk of pregnancy was not of primary significance. As one put it, 'Because people in care have such a shitty life they feel better if they're going to bed with someone' (Corlyon and McGuire 1997: 40).

Third, many people – particularly women – are faced with choices in which their responsibility for the health of other people and limited resources conflicts with what they know about healthy behaviour. A classic example is Oakley's (1989) evidence that pregnant women who smoke often see themselves as carrying out a coping strategy for dealing with stressors of various kinds, particularly when they lack adequate material resources. As one of Kempson's respondents put it, 'If my circumstances improved and I had less worry, I'd smoke less' (1996: 22). Oakley described this as an example of 'the rule that health-promoting work may be health-damaging for those who do it' (1989: 327). For some of Corlyon and McGuire's respondents, prioritising the health of others was reflected in their attitudes to abortion. 'I made the mistake so why should somebody else [the baby] suffer for what I've done' (1997: 64). Disadvantaged social circumstances also contributed to decisions to continue with pregnancies. As one young woman said, 'I thought, "Well what have I got to lose if I keep it? There's nowt else to do"' (Corlyon and McGuire 1997: 65).

Other evidence of Oakley's 'rule' can be seen in a variety of situations. For example, women on low incomes prioritised the needs of their male partners and their children for food, dealing with their own hunger and stress by getting by on cups of tea and cigarettes (Graham 1987). Parents who smoked also tried to protect their children from the financial costs of their smoking, for 'while low income smokers had poorer diets than non-smokers, there was no difference in the diets of their children' (Kempson 1996: 22). In a study of health and leisure in Hounslow, Asian women 'cited pressurised lives and a primary duty to serve their family' as key reasons for not exercising (Warren 1997: 26), and carers for adults have commonly provided care at the expense of physical, social and psychological damage to themselves (Anderson and Bury 1988; Atkin and Rollings 1996).

Fourth, structural factors can place health prevention and promotion outside the control of individuals. Roberts *et al.* (1993) found that parents' knowledge of environmental risks to their children in and outside homes on the Corkerhill estate in Glasgow was wider, more detailed and more specific than that of a group of professionals working in the area with some responsibility for accident prevention. While professionals were inclined to associate injuries with the characteristics of the families and to see education as a significant element in the solution, parents saw environmental hazards, such as gaps in balcony railings big enough for a baby to crawl through, hot water systems without thermostatic controls and lack of play space coupled with open access for cars, as accidents 'waiting to happen' (Roberts *et al.* 1993: 454). However, lack of resources (whether personal resources or resources available to the local authority) or the power to persuade others to take action meant that they experienced such hazards as out of their immediate control.

The interaction between individual and structural factors in health creation and maintenance was also revealed in Davison *et al.*'s (1992) study of lay attitudes to heart disease in South Wales: could apparently 'fatalistic' attitudes explain the failure of many to follow healthy lifestyle advice? Fatalism is the – implicitly wrong – assumption that control over a person's health, lies externally; or that, at least, they cannot exercise such control. On examination, respondents had identified three sets of factors as affecting the likelihood of heart disease. These were:

- personal differences between individuals, for example, due to heredity or upbringing;
- factors in the social environment, for example (1992: 679) 'relative wealth and access to resources, risks and dangers associated with occupation, loneliness'; and
- factors in the physical environment.

In addition, respondents reported examples of people who, for no apparent reasons, either behaved 'unhealthily' without the expected negative consequences, or else followed the rules but still got heart disease. They thus ascribed some element of chance or luck to the overall equation. However, this did not amount to a passive, irrational or culture-bound 'fatalism', so much as to a recognition of the limits of knowledge. Lay beliefs about health protection or promotion placed actions which they could take as individuals in the context of external influences over which they had little control. Davison *et al.* concluded (1992: 683): 'In our observation, popular belief and knowledge concerning the relationship of health to heredity, social conditions and the environment may be more in step with scientific epidemiology than the lifestyle-centred orientation of the health promotion world.'

HEALTH PROMOTION: A SUITABLE MODEL FOR HEALTH CREATION?

A limited analysis

A traditional professional model of health promotion is available.

However, we are not advocating that social work should adopt this, because of the dangers it embodies of compounding health inequalities. As the preceding two examples imply, health promotion messages have frequently targeted individual behaviour and given precedence to professional over lay understandings, without giving appropriate weight to the inequitable material and environmental circumstances and social forces in which lay efforts are enmeshed (DoH 1992). A focus on lifestyles and education remains persistently apparent in aspects of current government policies, despite its rhetoric (DoH 1998a). The programme of action to improve the health of children in the care system outlined in *Quality Protects* (DoH 1998d) targets measures for surveillance, immunisation and information-giving which will be of only limited benefit in the absence of action to improve the material and emotional circumstances and prospects of children in care and afterwards (Bywaters 1996). The development of Healthy Living Centres also shows evidence of a combination of welcome attention to promoting health amongst disadvantaged communities (such as older people, minority ethnic groups and those living in poverty), but with a continuing focus on individual behaviours (DoH 1998e).

This limitation in analysis feeds into health promotion policies and practices which can exacerbate inequalities in the chances of securing health. First, focusing excessively on individual behaviour can deflect attention from the more profound effects of wider social, economic and environmental circumstances. As described in Chapter 2, the material conditions of lay health work became more unequal in the UK during the 1980s and 1990s, with damaging consequences for many of the basic essentials of good health – income, housing, warmth, clean water, food, social support, and freedom from environmental hazards (Drakeford 1997; Ruane 1997; Standing 1997). The impact of business was also obscured, with the reluctance of the last government to impose 'unnecessary regulations' (DoH 1992: 106) on tobacco, alcohol and other industries finding echoes in the Labour Government's resistance to an early ban on tobacco sponsorship of Grand Prix motor races.

A second way in which health promotion and prevention can unwittingly exacerbate differences in health chances is if interventions, such as immunisation uptake (Reading *et al.* 1994) or health checks provided by GPs (Gillam 1992), are not equally accessed, or if they produce greater gains for those who are relatively better off (Blaxter 1990; Nettleton and Bunton 1995).

Third, health promotion and prevention approaches can incorporate institutionalised discrimination. The previous government's response to the emerging AIDS epidemic in the mid 1980s exemplifies this point. Homophobic and pro-family attitudes prevalent in the Tory party at the time reduced the effectiveness of both the public information campaign and the response of mainstream agencies (Watney 1996). Information was not effectively targeted at the gay community where the risk was greatest, while Section 28 of the Local Government Act blocked discussion of same-sex relationships in schools (and local authority residential homes) (King 1993).

Ahmad (1993) and Douglas (1996) have drawn attention to racist thinking underlying health promotion activities resulting in cultural pathologising, stereotyping and victim-blaming. For example, commentators have pointed out the absence from sex education materials provided by both public authorities and voluntary sector agencies of ethnic minority images and culturally appropriate content (Baxter 1994; Sanga, personal communication).

For many women on low incomes the legacy of individually focused health promotion material, urging, for example, healthy eating and active leisure pursuits, is responsibility without the power to exercise it. Oakley's rule (1989), discussed above, carries the implicit rider that the damage which can be caused by lay health promotion falls unfairly on women because, in most households, women hold primary responsibility for the welfare of male partners, of children and sometimes of other family members (Graham 1993).

Moreover, some health education messages have reinforced stereotypical ideas and images. One example was the Department of Health campaign against drink-driving which used, as a warning to drivers who drink, the image of a young disabled man in a wheelchair being fed by his mother.

NEW LABOUR: NEW POLICIES FOR HEALTH CREATION?

'Our Healthier Nation' (DoH 1998a) explicitly argued against such 'victim-blaming' approaches to health promotion and prevention. It proposed that responsibility for maximising population health is shared across sectors, with roles for central and local government, health authorities, business, voluntary bodies and individuals. It was argued that this 'involves a range of linked programmes including measures on welfare-to-work, crime, housing and education, as well as health' (DoH 1998a: 5). The approach was reflected in the subsequent announcement of 'national priorities' which emphasised 'tackling the root causes of ill health ... [including] fundamental inequalities in health' and 'breaking down barriers between services' (DoH 1998b: 3).

These twin objectives were repeated themes in the structural changes announced as the programme to modernise the NHS (DoH 1997a) and local government (Department of the Environment, Transport and the Regions (DETR) 1998a). Health Action Zones, based on local partnerships and covering at least the area of a Health Authority, were to 'achieve progress in addressing the causes of ill health and reducing health inequalities' (DoH 1997b: 1) 'linking the contribution of health and social services to work on regeneration, housing and employment' (DoH 1998b: 20), with about £50 million allocated to the first two 'waves' announced (DoH 1998f). Healthy Living Centres, funded through the New Opportunities Fund of the National Lottery, were also to be allocated £300 million 'to promote health, helping people of all ages to maximise their health and well-being, whatever their capacity for "fitness" in the traditional sense' (DoH 1997c:1). In each case the requirement of inter-agency partnership was coupled with an expectation that local people would be consulted, given opportunities to participate or be directly involved in project management.

Extended surveillance?

These 'new' forms of health promotion which emphasise community involvement and self-determination may seem more appropriate for social work, but contain their own dangers. They may increase inequalities in power, by extending forms of professional surveillance while generating increased opportunities for profit and exploitation (Bunton *et al.* 1995). Nettleton and Bunton (1995) argue that the concept of empowerment may reflect the appearance rather than the reality of redistribution of power and may hence institutionalise social divisions, producing acquiescence in inequitable, health-threatening conditions (Grace 1991; Wainwright 1996).

Moreover, the shift of health policy from treatment to prevention has been characterised as an extension of surveillance (Nettleton and Bunton 1995). The increased focus of attention on risk factors, particularly those which emphasise either behaviour (smoking, diet, physical activity) or the characteristics of a population (being socially excluded), extends the scope for intervention in two senses. First, it extends the areas of people's lives which are subject to the 'gaze' of health professionals or governments; second, it increases the proportion who are subject to surveillance, from those who are sick to those who might become sick (i.e. the total population).

A further consequence of such new public health policies is a shift from intermittent external surveillance by professionals to continuous self-surveillance. All aspects of 'lifestyle' come under scrutiny, from exercise to eating, from sex to stress management. A 'healthy' regime requires constant self-reflexive scrutiny of activities, intakes and internal reactions in response to myriad health messages. According to Nettleton and Bunton (1995: 53): 'From this perspective health promotion can be seen as one of many forms of contemporary governance which, through the establishment of appropriate social identities, forms a crucial dimension of effective social regulation.' The obligations of the citizen are not only to strive to become well if they fall sick, but to work not to become sick in the first place (Hepworth 1995). The disciplinary force is considerable, especially in a time of constrained public health and social care provision and insecurity of employment.

This extension of surveillance is also patterned by social inequalities. As Nettleton (1996) argues, women, as the main recipients of health care and the primary targets of health promotion policies, are particularly subject to surveillance. However, as Hann (1995: 37) points out: 'Although health advice is orientated towards women, it is the health and health needs of men and children that appear to be the goal of such activities.' Women also share with other groups – gay and lesbian people (Davies and Neal 1996); Black people (Watters 1996); elderly people (Ginn 1993) and disabled people (Shakespeare 1995) – the position of being seen as vulnerable, dangerous or a drain on resources (Castel 1991). This renders them the targets of health surveillance not necessarily in their interests.

A new role for social services?

Notwithstanding these concerns, a role in health creation for local authority and voluntary sector social services agencies, through an explicit agenda of tackling social disadvantage, is clearly signalled. As 'Our Healthier Nation' puts it:

> High quality social services play a vital role in the health of the people they serve. Decent support for older people, whether at home or in residential care; the protection and care of vulnerable children and young people; support for people with mental health problems; and helping people with disabilities live more independent lives: health and social care are often one and the same. By protecting the vulnerable, caring for those with problems and supporting people back into independence and dignity, social services have a vital role in fostering better health.
>
> (DoH 1998a: 23)

However, as we turn now to examine social work's record on health creation and the potential for the future, we will argue that a substantial change in the awareness, attitudes and actions of social workers and social work agencies is necessary if this potential is to be realised.

SOCIAL WORK AND HEALTH CREATION

Almost all aspects of social work provision can be seen as relevant to the essential needs which underpin health creation. Income enhancement, securing appropriate accommodation, the provision of social care resources and services, bringing oppressive conditions to public notice, enabling children and adults to be free from violence, abuse and self-harm, and opposing institutionalised oppression all contribute to better health. However, many users of services report alienating experiences of rationing, stigma and loss of control (Becker 1997). The second half of this chapter considers limitations to social work's contribution, but also how it can promote health creation on a more equitable basis. This will be done by examining examples of social work's role in relation to the primary conditions for more equal chances of creating or maintaining health:

- securing basic material resources;
- improving physical environments; and
- developing more just social environments.

Securing basic material resources

At the heart of lay people's efforts to develop and maintain good health is the need for an adequate basic income. Kempson describes the multiple health-related consequences for individuals and families in hardship who are doing without 'luxuries' and a social life, cutting back on – or going without – essentials:

> The struggle to make ends meet not only affects family life, but can result in poor diet, lack of fuel and water, poor housing, and homelessness, debt, poor physical health, and stress and mental health problems. The poorer people are, the more likely they are to experience these problems.
>
> (Kempson 1996: 30)

Sometimes family ties are threatened when debts cannot be paid or family commitments, such as providing a wreath for a funeral, cannot be met. Constant money problems and the absence of relief gained from going out or contact with friends make for turbulent social relationships and sometimes violence (Kempson 1996). It is therefore not surprising that, from its origins, involvement with social work has been inextricably linked to poverty, though not always to the benefit of service users.

Social services departments: Part of the problem?

Throughout the 1980s and 1990s, a key element in the creation of greater inequalities in income in the UK was the government's attempt to restrict expenditure on the social security system (Beresford and Croft 1995; Craig 1992). This objective was pursued by a variety of mechanisms, including benefits either failing to keep pace with earnings or being cut, tighter eligibility criteria, stigmatising, inefficient and off-putting processes and continuing low take-up. Moreover, government policies also enhanced the role of state social work in controlling public expenditure on income maintenance. Becker (1997) charted the significance for social services departments of two key measures: the social fund and revised community care arrangements. In each case, entitlements backed by unlimited budgets – to grants for exceptional needs on the one hand and for care provided free at the point of delivery, either from the NHS or through the social security system, on the other – were replaced by rationed access to capped budgets. In the first case, social services departments successfully resisted close involvement in administering the social fund; in the second, desire for a central role in community care prevailed.

Becker (1997) has outlined four key criticisms of social services departments' responses to these developments. First, departments and social workers were seen to distance themselves from anti-poverty work – except where charging created the incentive for income maximisation. A reluctance to be seen as agents of the social security system in managing the social fund, coupled with pressures from increasing demand, capped resources and negative publicity from child deaths inquiries, led to an increasing tendency to see poverty as an inevitable backdrop to practice, the province of other workers and other agencies, rather than the subject of active intervention. This went hand in hand with the emergence of anti-oppressive practice strategies in which issues of class and material inequality were often sidelined, despite reports which showed that poverty remained the single factor most widely associated with social work contact (see Chapter 1). Thus, despite Tree's (1997) claim that social service workers were the major advice service in relation to disability benefits, large numbers of disabled people failed to claim their entitlements, while Age Concern estimated that £1.6 billion a year went unclaimed by older people (Whiteley 1997; see also French 1995).

Second, even where departments had resources of direct value to families in poverty – such as direct payments to disabled people, Section 17 grants for children 'in need', Section 21 payments to asylum seekers, payments to care leavers and foster carers (including extended family members) and services such as meals on wheels, luncheon clubs and day care – these were often deployed inequitably and without a sense of their strategic significance in combating poverty (Local Government Anti-Poverty Unit 1996a). Criticisms have included variations between and within authorities in levels of funding available and the range of goods on which they could be spent; a lack of clear allocation policies and criteria; inadequate publicity; and a failure to effectively monitor expenditure and its outcomes. These have resulted in the government's intention to institute a national standard for charging for community care, the 'Fair Access to Care' initiative (DoH 1998c).

Third, a parallel set of criticisms has been levelled at charging systems (Balloch and Robertson 1995; Harvey and Robertson 1995). Local authorities could not be held responsible for the geographical inequity which resulted from the blanket expectation that 9 per cent of community care costs would be obtained through charges, whatever the social make-up of the district. However, the development of local charging systems has resulted in wide variations in the scope and structure of charges, in approaches to means testing and in practices such as systems for representation, review and appeal.

Fourth, social services departments have been criticised for failing to challenge the contradictions and perverse incentives arising from the interaction of different pieces of legislation (Tree 1997). For example, the principles of the Children Act 1989 with regard to continuing parental responsibility for, and involvement with, children are at odds with aspects of social security legislation, which immediately reduces a lone parent's income when her child is accommodated, and is unable to reallocate benefits when care is shared between parents.

While social services departments alone could not compensate for the extensive levels of income inequality to be found nationally, the absence of *strategy* for maximising the beneficial impact of resources and minimising the effects of charging on the poverty of service users is significant. It is particularly disappointing that social services departments have often had limited engagement with the anti-poverty strategies which have emerged in local authorities in the past ten years (Fimister 1994; Local Government Anti-Poverty Unit 1996b). Becker (1997) identified five key elements of such strategies:

- targeted anti-poverty interventions focusing on particular groups or defined areas;
- the decentralisation of services, sometimes involving devolution of power;
- economic and community regeneration, often linking anti-poverty strategies to broader urban regeneration;
- income maintenance and maximisation, incorporating welfare rights and debt advice and policies on benefits administered by local authorities; and
- charging policies, including rebates and exemptions.

These policies have generated many local initiatives, including take-up campaigns and other forms of income maximisation, better access to welfare rights advice and debt counselling, the creation of partnerships through which credit unions, LETS schemes and co-operatives have been developed, and broad initiatives for economic and social regeneration, often involving European Union funding. However, social services department involvement has been largely absent.

There is also little evidence that social services departments in general have been significantly involved in economic regeneration programmes such as City Challenge and Single Regeneration Budget projects – not that these initiatives are a panacea (Mayo 1997). Social services have an interest in economic regeneration in three respects: to meet service users' needs; as large employers; and as regulators and purchasers of private sector residential and community-based care services. They could have had an active role in encouraging employment and in setting standards concerning pay and working conditions in what has traditionally been a low-paid, low-investment, predominantly female labour market.

If social workers and social services agencies persist in ignoring the evidence from service users that assistance in dealing with poverty and its effects is often their dominant concern (Davis and Wainwright 1996), and fail to construct and support strategies which can at least mitigate the pervasive effects of poverty on health, they will continue to be avoided and mistrusted by their clients, for whom involvement with 'social services and social work has become fraught with danger – part of the problem of daily living, rather than part of the solution' (Becker 1997: 89).

Re-discovering poverty work: Voluntary sector initiatives, collectivism and campaigning

Outside social services departments there is some evidence of a 're-discovery' of poverty within social work. The British Association of Social Workers launched a national anti-poverty strategy at its annual general meeting in 1997, while many major voluntary sector social work organisations have shown an increasing desire to tackle poverty directly through economic measures that target specific populations or localities. This is in addition to the more traditional routes of welfare advice, debt counselling and the direct provision of subsidised meals and access to resources such as washing-machines and leisure activities (Cohen and Wiffen 1996).

Voluntary sector organisations have become involved in boosting collective financial resources in poorer neighbourhoods through the development of credit unions. Backed by organisations such as Oxfam (Johnson and Rogaly 1997) and Barnardos (Drakeford and Hudson 1994) as one aspect of world-wide microfinance anti-poverty schemes, credit unions are now about 600 strong in England and Wales and number about 200,000 members (HM Treasury 1998a), concentrated in areas with high levels of deprivation. Initiated by community workers, they provide affordable credit to members, based on regular savings of small amounts in schemes whose assets and organisation are managed co-operatively (Hudson *et al.* 1994). Free life insurance on savings is also available and repayments are organised at levels which previous savings indicate are manageable (Hudson *et al.* 1994; Johnson and Rogaly 1997). Members may otherwise be unable to access high-street credit due to discrimination on grounds of low income, location or ethnic minority identity (Herbert and Kempson 1996).

Credit unions have their limitations and shortcomings. They do not challenge the legitimacy of harshly divisive, health-threatening economic structures. They can fail to incorporate the very poorest residents in a locality, who lack the means to save even small sums regularly (Kempson 1994). Nevertheless, there is case-study evidence of members in relative poverty benefiting in many ways. Repairs and purchases which are crucial to maintaining well-being, involving fridges, cookers and washing-machines, have become affordable. The material costs of being able to participate in landmark social events such as birthdays and Christmas have been covered. Unforeseen expenditure has been prevented from precipitating a morass of debt at exorbitant rates of interest to 'loan sharks', with potentially dire secondary consequences such as eviction (Hudson *et al.* 1994; Johnson and Rogaly 1997; Newtown/South Aston Credit Union Ltd 1997). What credit unions make available – affordable credit – is a financial resource associated with improved chances of achieving levels of physical and psychological well-being which more affluent sections of the population take for granted.

Another example from outside the traditional voluntary social work sector is the Big Step programme which has grown out of *The Big Issue*, a business venture designed to provide homeless people with the chance of an income through selling *The Big Issue* magazine (*The Big Issue* 1997). Big Step aims to provide homeless people with the opportunity of moving on into more substantial employment by providing access to job opportunities, training, health care and accommodation. Its key features are that in conjunction with a caseworker, the *Big Issue* vendor constructs a twelve-month resettlement strategy. Vendors becomes purchasers of the services they want, through direct access to funding, the aim being to ensure that control is in their own hands. In return, vendors must agree 'to do everything they can to achieve the strategy ... [including] turning up on time for interviews ... [and] maintaining tenancy agreements' (*The Big Issue in the North* 1997: 4).

Alongside these collective forms of action to shore up the material resources available to specific populations or localities are examples of campaigning for changes in the wider system. One case in point is older people's action on relative poverty. The National Pensions' Convention was founded in 1979 and has a million and a half affiliated members. The cornerstone of its central aim of social justice for older people is a decent level of income (Ginn 1993) and it has a rolling programme of campaigning, lobbying and demonstrations to this end (Midlands Pensioner Convention 1993 and 1996). This secured an important victory for more equal chances of health maintenance when it turned the Conservative government's 1993 attempt to impose Value Added Tax (VAT) at 17.5 per cent on domestic heating fuel into a highly contentious public issue. Outright abolition was not secured, but the rate was halved to 8 per cent (Midlands Pensioner Convention 1993; *Sunday Mirror* 4 July 1993, 17 October 1993 and 5 December 1993). Direct action by the Disabled Action Network also won prominence in late 1997 as part of the campaign by disabled people and their supporters against possible cuts in benefits and the programme of review of existing entitlements. The wider government agenda of a weakened commitment to a comprehensive, state, insurance-based social security system has apparently not been deflected, but subsequent delays in announcements of fundamental changes in social security policy suggest that an important shot was fired across the bows of privatisation.

Improving physical environments

The activities just described constitute the opening up of areas of social work practice not currently recognised as central, although germane to health creation and maintenance. Concern with the physical environment also requires a change of emphasis in practice.

The environmental agenda

Links between health creation and a sustainable environment are increasingly being made at international, national and local levels of policy-making. The World Health Organisation's Ottowa Charter contained the pledge 'to counteract the pressures towards harmful products, resources depletion, unhealthy living conditions and environments, and bad nutrition; and to focus attention on public health issues such as pollution, occupational hazards, housing and settlements' (cited in Jones and Sidell 1997: 108). Campaigning organisations like Friends of the Earth (1995) also argue that economic development threatens the quality of the most basic requirements for health: water, air and food. Meanwhile, outside formal organisations, environmental activists use direct action techniques to publicise the health-damaging effects of developments such as the extension of polluting road and air transport systems and food production methods which rely on genetic engineering, chemicals and intensive livestock management (Friends of the Earth 1995).

This focus of activity may seem to be beyond the scope or objectives of social work. However, social services agencies cannot avoid environmental impact, although they have tended to avoid explicit engagement with the issue. For example, social services organisations are already involved with diet and nutrition, directly purchasing and/or providing food for hundreds of thousands of people through residential care, day centres, luncheon clubs and meals on wheels services. As such they are large customers of the food industry, with potential leverage. They spend substantial sums of money on providing or supporting private transport, which contributes to pollution; use large amounts of paper and other equipment which could be recycled; and, as significant players in pension funds worth billions of pounds, could influence investment policies. Social services and voluntary sector agencies also have the possibility of engaging with these issues through programmes such as the WHO 'Healthy Cities' initiatives which were given a strong green dimension by the Rio Earth Summit's Agenda 21. Local authorities in the UK now have a statutory duty to produce Agenda 21 plans which emphasise community involvement and cross-agency partnerships (Thornton and Hams 1996). As in the case of poverty, the first call in relation to the physical environment is not to develop new provision but for an awareness of the impact of existing policies and practices and a strategic approach to the deployment of resources to reduce rather than contribute to health inequalities (Hoff 1997). This is exemplified in the case of policy and practice relating to housing provision and accidents, discussed next.

Housing

Alongside, and inextricably linked to, financial poverty, housing is a major concern in many service users' lives (Davis and Wainwright 1996). More equal access to safe, secure, affordable and comfortable accommodation is a *sine qua non* of reducing inequalities in health, because it is a prerequisite to securing basic income and work; because of the stresses associated with poor housing and their impact on relationships; and because insanitary, cold, damp and dangerous physical conditions have direct effects on health (Barnardos [no date]; Barrow and Bachan 1997; Khan 1997; Llewellin and Murdock 1996; Means *et al.* 1997).

There are many overlapping dimensions of social work involvement with housing issues encompassing work with homeless people and those in temporary accommodation; contribution to the provision of adapted housing for some disabled people; partnerships in the provision of and access to supported and sheltered accommodation and adult placements in the community; and the provision and purchase of residential care. In addition, the impact of overcrowding, damp and disrepair, as well as the damaging effects of accidents, harassment (including racial harassment), crime and the fear of crime in disadvantaged areas have negative consequences for many social work service users (for useful summaries of recent research and policy developments see the Joseph Rowntree Foundation *Findings* and *Foundations* pamphlets).

The record of social services departments' response to housing needs is mixed, often lacking a strategic dimension. Stewart and Stewart (1993: 17) found that 'help (with housing problems) is particularly appreciated' but that 'social workers find housing problems among the most difficult to handle'. The service offered in 90 per cent of cases in successive studies was 'perfunctory advice and information and the case was closed within a week, usually the same day' (1993: 18). Stewart and Stewart argue that lack of awareness of the significance of housing problems in service users' lives, perhaps resulting from familiarity, coupled with the view that housing is someone else's problem, lead to social workers either ignoring the issue or adopting pathologising attitudes which compound the problem. While there are many examples of good practice, these tend to be patchy (making services an inequitable, geographical lottery) and are often special projects rather than mainstream activity (Means *et al.* 1997; Joseph Rowntree Foundation 1995).

Once again, it is frequently social work in voluntary sector agencies which provides examples of positive practice, encompassing research, campaigning, direct service provision and community development. NCH Action for Children's 'House Our Youth 2000' campaign was developed before the 1997 election to call for government action to combat the impact of homelessness on rising numbers of young people (Mead 1997). In the absence of official statistics, estimates of young people who were homeless in 1996 varied from 33,000 to 246,000 (Dunn and McClusky 1997). The withdrawal of benefit from most 16–17-year-olds in 1988, replaced by a place on a Youth Training Scheme and access to short-term 'severe hardship' payments, has left increasing numbers with inadequate income for subsistence, let alone housing. Research conducted for the government by MORI found that 'a quarter of severe hardship claimants had needed to beg, steal or sell drugs in order to survive. This proportion rose to a half of those who had been living rough' (cited in Allard and Dunn 1997: 4). Meanwhile, the enforced reliance of greater numbers of young people on their families of origin for continued accommodation, due to a combination of policy changes brought in by the previous government, has rendered them vulnerable to 'push factors' including violence, abuse, family breakdown, being thrown out or asked to leave to ease family poverty (Smith *et al.* 1998).

Voluntary sector agencies are also working to counteract shortcomings in statutory child-care policy and practice, largely reflecting funding shortfalls (which contribute to and compound the hardship associated with housing problems after young people leave care), by commissioning and publishing research. For example, nearly half the care leavers surveyed by Save the Children (1995) had received no leaving-care grant while, for others, grants varied from £5 to £1,800. Garnett (1992) found 25 per cent of care leavers were not receiving any support from social services within nine months of leaving care. Voluntary agencies' own practice is also not flawless. Carlen (1994) has shown that their initiatives can compound exclusion from key resources through failing to address specific requirements; for example, denying access to disabled potential residents; imposing unrealistic admissions criteria such as not admitting people with mental health problems who are also drug users, and imposing unrealistically strict behaviour codes for residents. Even if rehousing is achieved, it is not clear to what extent this is sustained, nor how far it cancels out the long-term social and physical and psychological disadvantage that has accrued in the care system (Fisher and Collins 1993). Nevertheless, voluntary sector initiatives, by opening up access to accommodation, employment and social support and by attempting to incorporate users' direction of personal programmes, may provide the linchpins of improved chances of health and well-being (Centrepoint 1997).

Accidents and the built environment

Health hazards in the physical environment resulting in increased chances of accidental death and injury are particularly likely to disadvantage social work service users. Cars are a prime example. As Erskine (1996: 154, 155) argues:

> those who are in groups least likely to benefit from the use of cars [women, children, older people, people living in poverty, disabled people] are disproportionately likely to be victims of fatal road accidents ... [Moreover] those who are not direct beneficiaries of current car-oriented transport policies are likely to experience a high incidence of accident risk, albeit at a time when the overall rate of injury in accidents is decreasing.

Williams *et al.* (1996) found that the strong negative association of social class with death rates from accidents was not apparent in the numbers of injuries which resulted in contacts with GPs or hospitals. However, types of accident and their treatment were strongly patterned by class, with better-off children more likely to be injured as a result of relatively expensive leisure activities – even though they were more likely to be using safety equipment – and as passengers in cars, while children of less affluent parents were more likely to be injured in other people's houses and on the streets as pedestrians. Working-class children were more likely to be admitted to hospital (and miss time from school) but, as this did not correlate with greater severity of injuries, Williams suggests it reflected health professionals' lack of confidence in parents' care.

Despite the repeated official recommendation of increased education to prevent accidents in general, lack of knowledge of risk is not the major problem (Carter and Jones 1993; Graham and Firth 1992; Green 1995; Roberts *et al.* 1993). The main issues to be tackled are the circumstances – primarily poverty – which place people in environments with greater risk and poorly designed living spaces (McNeish and Roberts 1995). Parents' suggestions to a Barnardos' survey included: 'clearing away the glass and dog dirt', 'knocking down derelict buildings', 'more police to make sure people don't start fires in the empty houses', 'a fence round the brook' and 'soft floors in playgrounds' (McNeish and Roberts 1995: 20–1).

For mainstream social work, it is non-accidental injury which has dominated the child-care agenda with the focus of practice increasingly on the investigation and regulation of families rather than providing appropriate support (Parton 1997). The fact that the rate of death in childhood from 'accidents' – including those associated with poor-quality housing and the built environment (Roberts and Power 1996) – runs at about fifteen times the rate of deaths associated with non-accidental injury (Woodrofe *et al.* 1993) has never been a central issue for 'child protection' strategies.

Developing more just social environments

In a similar pattern to the social work response to inequalities in material resources and the physical environment, inequalities in the risk of violence and self-harm, beyond child abuse, constitute key features of the health-damaging social environment. These have been infrequently addressed in mainstream social work and rarely on the basis of preventive strategies.

Violence: A significant risk to health

The four UK Women's Aid Federations, in conjunction with allies and counterparts world-wide, have shown that domestic violence, specifically men's violence to their women partners or ex-partners (Morley and Mullender 1994), is a widespread, socially constructed health risk for women. Such violence has been shown as likely to be experienced by 25–30 per cent of women (Mooney 1994; Painter 1991). The degree of physical injury sustained has been documented as commonly severe, with the severity escalating once violence starts (Dobash and Dobash 1980). Psychological injuries range from the destruction of self-esteem and self-confidence to lifetimes lived in terror (Mullender 1996). Analysis of the origins of this violence has revealed it to be legitimated by ideologies of male dominance (Dobash and Dobash 1992); by the continued absence of comprehensive legislation and refuge funding; and by the unreliability of public agencies' support (Hague and Malos 1994). Gendered inequalities in income, employment, housing and child-care have been demonstrated to reinforce women's vulnerability (Dobash and Dobash 1992).

While the high incidence of violence persists, key institutions are being influenced to develop policies which not only facilitate women's escape from it (Dobash and Dobash 1992) but which focus on men's responsibility to end it. Across the 1990s, police forces in

England and Wales have taken measures to increase the number of incidents of domestic violence recorded and treated as crimes (Mullender 1996). Meanwhile, local authorities have started backing zero tolerance campaigns (Mullender 1996). While the issue is still marginalised in social services departments' day-to-day practice, attempts are being made to be alert to and respond more swiftly to the problem. Through collaboration with the Womens Aid Federations, social services department (SSD) workers are becoming better informed about women's legal rights and about local resources. Specialist liaison responsibilities with local refuges have been instituted. There is evidence that women from refuges are now approaching SSDs in greater confidence and being met with a more informed and swifter response with important implications for their health (Mullender and Humphreys 1998).

A concerted campaign against homophobic violence has developed more recently than action against domestic violence, but again an initiative aiming to uncover and publicise endemic violence grounded in social inequalities has sprung from self-help activism rather than from professionals. In the absence of official statistics (Mason and Palmer 1996), Stonewall, a civil rights campaigning organisation which has developed from the lesbian, gay and bisexual rights movement (Stonewall 1996a), co-ordinated the first national survey of homophobic crime and harassment in 1994. Distributed through Stonewall's own database and via gay publications and lesbian/gay mailing lists, the survey yielded approximately 4,200 replies incorporating several hundred detailed accounts (Stonewall 1996b). The degree and extent of violence revealed and its health consequences are shocking. Of all respondents, 34 per cent of men and 24 per cent of women had experienced violence in the last five years because of their sexuality. One in six had been 'hit, punched or kicked' (Mason and Palmer 1996: 7); 32 per cent had been harassed. Most assaults were perpetrated by strangers, but such incidents also occurred at home and work. Of those attacked, 25 per cent needed medical attention, 18 per cent needed time off work and 79 per cent suffered stress or fear (Mason and Palmer 1996).

The conjunction of different dimensions of disadvantage increased the chances of violence. Forty per cent of Asian, 45 per cent of African Caribbean and 50 per cent of disabled respondents had experienced homophobic violence (Mason and Palmer 1996). Younger people were particularly vulnerable: 48 per cent had experienced violence and 61 per cent had been harassed. Of these violent attacks, 40 per cent took place at school, with 50 per cent of the perpetrators being fellow students.

> 'I am 17 years old and am openly gay in the small town of Crewe that I live in. Throughout my school life, I have been beaten up, mugged and even threatened with knives more times than I care to mention. The long-term effects of the violence I face is worse though. I don't often go out on my own anywhere now.'
>
> (Mason and Palmer 1996: 20)

In the face of such widespread and vicious violence, there is evidence that campaigning efforts are nevertheless beginning to influence opinion and policy. Many lesbian and gay police liaison groups have set up violence monitoring schemes (Cosis Brown 1998). However, there is little evidence of parallel strategic responses within mainstream social services. Only by redressing the marginalisation of gay, lesbian and bisexual rights as a social work issue may social work cease to be 'part of the problem' rather than part of the solution to this health threat (Cosis Brown 1998).

Self-harm and suicide

Self-harm, including suicide, is another widespread, socially constructed health hazard in which statutory social work agencies generally have shown little interest. The incidence is substantial in Britain: suicide accounts for nearly 6,500 deaths a year and hospital referrals alone suggest there are approximately 100,000 attempted suicides annually (Samaritans 1997a). In a ground-breaking study across twenty-four localities, Gunnell *et al.* (1995) demonstrated strong relationships between suicide, parasuicide, psychiatric morbidity and socio-economic deprivation. Further dimensions to the ways in which suicide and parasuicide may be patterned by social inequalities have been drawn out by other studies. Raleigh *et al.* (1990) and Raleigh and Balarajan (1992) found that across the 1970s and early 1980s the level of suicide rates among Indian women immigrants aged 15–24, most of whom were married, was about twice as high as the general rate for women in Britain of corresponding ages. Surveys estimate that approximately one in five lesbians, young gay men and bisexuals attempt suicide (Mason and Palmer 1996). Suicide rates among young men aged 15–24 years old rose by 75 per cent during the mid- to late 1980s (Wilkinson 1996a) and have been shown to be associated with the acceleration of unemployment and growing restrictions on benefits (Wilkinson 1994b).

While mainstream social work generally has been involved in suicide and self-harm as a mental health issue, working after the event to reduce repeat attempts, the Samaritans have achieved national recognition for the development of helplines. With only a small paid staff and relying almost exclusively on volunteers, the Samaritans have run a round-the-clock, confidential, primarily telephone-based counselling service for people who are 'suicidal or despairing' and are the major preventitive service (Samaritans 1997a). The scale of the take-up rate for this service is sobering. In 1995, 3,878,000 contacts were made (Samaritans 1997a) – an increase of 29 per cent in ten years (Samaritans 1997b). There is some evidence (Lester 1994) that the growth in the number of Samaritan centres is associated with a reduction in suicide rates by gassing, stabbing and piercing. Confirmatory evidence that a large number of callers view the Samaritans as a last line of defence against suicide is provided by the organisation's own findings. Approximately a third of the three million annual calls are silent. Of the remainder, 25 per cent specifically express suicidal thoughts (Samaritans 1997a). When the Samaritans set up an email network (embodying a confidential facility) as a means of communication appealing to young men, 80 per cent of the 526 callers in the first six months acknowledged they had suicidal feelings (Samaritans 1997b).

The one and a half million calls to the Samaritans not explicitly focusing on suicide may, of course, incorporate this as an unexpressed preoccupation. A content breakdown of calls is not available (research officer, Samaritans, personal communication). However, their high incidence suggests that the Samaritans may be fulfilling a more primary preventative role in suicide through also relieving emotional isolation arising from unequal social relations. Relative deprivation has been shown to be associated with reduced chances of access to supportive social networks and subsequently with poorer chances of psychological well-being (Blaxter 1990). Moreover, theoretically 'close' personal relationships in our society, with partners, family, parents and even intimate friends, have been revealed as a site of social division embodying sexist, ageist, class-ridden, homophobic, racist and disablist behaviours, and hence not necessarily good for emotional care. The intervention of mental health care professionals may compound such conditions (McLeod 1994). Therefore it seems possible that it is because discriminatory and hierarchical social relations are failing to meet people's emotional needs that they are turning in such large numbers to the Samaritans.

For their part the Samaritans are taking steps to equalise access to their services. Touch-text telephone lines have been introduced for deaf and hearing-impaired callers and banks of volunteers speaking languages other than English are being organised. Outreach initiatives are being set up, such as the distribution of charge-cards with the Samaritans' telephone number to schoolchildren and homeless young people, supplemented by contact volunteers available at drop-in centres (outreach worker, Samaritans, personal communication). Meanwhile, the initiative of callers in ringing the Samaritans in such large numbers remains a testimony to the distorted nature of our social relations: the best chance of help with the most profound emotional problems is frequently identified as coming from someone you have never met.

CONCLUSION

The significance of action for health creation and maintenance is profound and long lasting, affecting not only present but future generations. Like the Black Report (DHSS 1980), the Acheson Report emphasised the long-term impact of influences laid down in childhood.

> Small size or thinness at birth are associated with coronary heart disease, diabetes and hypertension in later life. As two principal determinants of a baby's weight at birth are the mother's pre-pregnant weight and her own birthweight, the need for policies to improve the health of (future) mothers and their children is obvious.
>
> (Independent Inquiry 1998: 9)

However, the impact of 'cumulative environmental insults' – and the benefits of intervention – continue throughout the life course (Davey Smith *et al.* 1998c)

Of course, social work cannot, on its own, change either the global economic conditions or the diverse forms of oppressive social relations which affect children and adults of all ages, but there is evidence in this chapter that social work by no means maximises its opportunities to have a positive impact on health creation, and can even be 'part of the problem'. Nevertheless, social work whih is permeated by the objective of reducing inequalities, which acts locally in strategic alliances in the framework of a broader analysis, can contribute to creating better conditions for health.

Chapter 4

Ill health at home

INTRODUCTION

In this chapter, we focus on addressing social work's impact on inequalities in ill health. In describing how the experience of ill health is permeated by socially created inequalities we first highlight the perspective of lay health workers (Stacey 1988), looking at both people who are ill and those closely involved with them, and the twin processes of giving and receiving care (Aronson 1998). Second, we examine negative aspects of current forms of social work practice, and finally, we discuss forms of practice which can reduce inequalities and promote a better quality of life for people who are living with illness.

Lay health work against the odds

Serious acute or long-term ill health are amongst the most significant of life experiences, while long-term illness is widespread (Gray 1993; Woodrofe *et al.* 1993). Moreover, not only have rates of GP consultation increased between 1981–2 and 1991–2 but 'the people seen are more severely ill than a decade ago' (Editorial 1995: 284*)*. Successive General Household Surveys recorded that the incidence of self-defined 'long-standing limiting illness'[2] (LLI) in children almost doubled between 1975 and 1994, when one child in eleven between 5 and 15 was affected (Cooper *et al.* 1998a). By the age of 45 almost 30 per cent of adults report a LLI. For those over 75 this rises to 50 per cent (Sidell 1995).

The chances of experiencing serious illness are permeated by social inequality (see Chapter 2). Social inequalities take physical form, are embodied in unjust, unnecessary pain, exhaustion and malaise: 'Our bodies are a site of oppressive social relations' (Bywaters and McLeod 1996a: 16). Once serious ill health is experienced, as we show in detail in the course of this chapter, further socially constructed inequalities cluster around, affecting, for example, chances of achieving good-quality treatment and care. The socially constructed nature of inequalities in ill health also means that actual or potential users of social work services are disproportionately likely to suffer significant ill health and inequalities in treatment and care. However, discussion of physical illness as a factor resulting directly or indirectly in social work involvement or as a focus for anti-oppressive practice is rarely found in social work discourse in the UK (McLeod and Bywaters 1999).

Most ill health is grappled with while people are living in their own homes and away from the attention and care of health (or social care) professionals. Though brief stays in hospital, consultations in surgeries, day hospitals or outpatients clinics and prescribed treatments will all still be highly significant events, much of the management of illness, including looking after yourself or others, working for recovery, putting up with symptoms and taking home and commercial remedies, is undertaken without recourse to medical advice or intervention (Popay 1992). Hannay (1980) found that even when respondents rated their symptoms as severe, over a quarter did not seek medical treatment. And when people do consult doctors, action taken by the 'patient' is usually crucial to successful recovery (Conrad 1985; Eiser *et al.* 1995), while long-term medical conditions, by definition, resist the curative efforts of medicine.

A range of social factors contribute to – or undermine – the quality of life of people who face serious or long-term illness and aid – or prevent – recovery. Repeatedly, researchers have found that it is not the severity of the physical condition, the demands of the treatment, or the frequency or length of attendance at hospital which determine the sense of well-being or the quality of life of patients and supporters, but a variety of material, environmental and social resources which are not equally distributed (Ahmad and Atkin 1996; Anderson 1992; Anderson and Bury 1988; Barlow *et al.* 1998; Beresford *et al.* 1996; Charles and Walters 1998; Joseph Rowntree *Findings* 1997, 1998a and 1998b; Sloper 1996). Differences in income and wealth between patients and carers of different socio-economic groups are compounded by assumptions based on gender, racial, disablist and heterosexist stereotypes – for example, that women are 'natural' carers; black people 'look after their own'; disabled people are necessarily dependent on others; gay men and les-bians have less committed relationships; and poor health is an inevitable accompaniment of old age.

Inequalities in ill health and disability

Our perspective proceeds from a social model of health which focuses on the impact of social inequalities on health chances and experience. This parallels and complements the arguments advanced by the disability rights movement. We see the totality of bodily experience as socially constructed and subject to the impact of social inequalities. This includes the creation and maintenance of health, entry into ill-health, the physical and emotional dimensions to ill-health and recovery or death. We, therefore, address aspects of the impact of social inequalities on health and ill-health fromwhich the disability rights movement – in focusing on the impact of disablist external factors on enduring physical impairment and rightly rejecting the construction of the experience as a 'medical' issue – has drawn away attention.

One consequence of our approach is to bridge the divide between the discourses on inequalities in health and ill health and on disability as constituting socially constructed disadvantage (Barnes and Mercer 1996). First, from our standpoint, the concept of 'disablism' is as germane to the experience of ill health as to impairment. Laungani's (1992) account of his own serious illness not only describes experiencing dimensions of physical suffering previously invisible to him, but also reflects the pervasiveness of disablist notions of physical impairment equalling worthlessness.

> My strength had ebbed to such a low level that it was virtually impossible for me to squeeze out toothpaste from a tube, turn on the taps in my bath or even hold a mug of tea in my hand. I felt weak, incapable, useless.
>
> (Laungani 1992: 23)

Second, we regard the experience of physical impairment not simply as socially constructed by disablist responses to it but as bearing the impact of other dimensions of social disadvantage: class, 'race', gender, age and sexual orientation. Third, as reflected in this chapter, we consider a rights perspective characterising the disability movement also to be critical to the dimensions of ill health that we discuss.

We next illustrate how illness is permeated by socially created inequalities by discussing three aspects of the experience of illness which should be a focus of social workers' attention:

- entry to ill health;
- initial access to NHS services; and
- the distribution of social and material resources.

While examining the experience of ill health from the perspective of lay health workers, our analysis is grounded in a 'broader politics of health care' (Annandale 1998: 30): how social divisions, mediated through social structures, policies and practices, are reflected in the individual experience of illness.

ILL HEALTH: AN EXPERIENCE OF INEQUALITY AND DISCRIMINATION

Entry to ill health

The process of identifying ill health almost invariably begins with lay people. However, at all ages there is an unequal distribution, not only of responsibilities, but also of opportunities for identifying illness. Parents feel that they sometimes lack sufficient information on which to base judgements about whether to consult a doctor (Kai 1996), and such information is unevenly available, especially for those for whom written sources, in either a second or a first language, or via the Internet, are not accessible (Greenhalgh *et al.* 1998). Children, young people and adults who are homeless, socially isolated, live alone or in residential care and lack the close attention and concern of another adult may also lack the sources of lay advice which usually precede doctors' appointments (Bywaters 1996). Disablist barriers to communication or assessment of symptoms are also present. For example, the primary health care system 'largely relies on a person's ability to recognise and report symptoms of ill health', according to Rodgers (1994: 13), who adds: 'People with learning disabilities may have difficulty with this.' Both formal and informal carers may fail to listen, or not perceive this as their role. High levels of untreated ill health result (Gaze 1998; Howells 1986).

Where symptoms are identified, the onset of ill health cannot be simplistically read as a personal tragedy; it is an event heavily patterned by attendant social circumstances. For example, Pound *et al.* (1998) interviewed forty men and women living in the East End of London some ten months after a stroke. The stroke had had considerable impact on their lives: on their ability – unassisted – to leave the house, get around the neighbourhood, do housework and pursue leisure activities; on their speech and self-care; on their memories, sense of identity, relationships with others and with themselves and their bodies. 'However, the idea of a happy "before" and a tragic "after", in which the stroke brought a bright and active life to a sudden halt, was reported by two interviewees only' (Pound *et al.* 1998: 495).

The stroke entered lives characterised by crises and hardship. 'Mr Victor' from the Caribbean was living in hunger and poverty. Two Bangladeshi men were living in totally unsuitable housing conditions. Twenty-five people also mentioned pre-existing health conditions. For some the stroke merely compounded existing problems, for others it paled into insignificance beside other problems faced. The pain, suffering and death they faced were inextricably connected to other dimensions of socially created inequality.

The care with which people manage the disclosure of information about their illness also reflects widespread discriminatory reactions (Davey and Seale 1996). In 'public' accounts (Cornwell 1984), people may deny the existence of illness altogether (Carricaburu and Pierret 1995, concerning HIV); deny the diagnosis, for example, describing themselves as 'a bit chesty' rather than as asthmatic (Adams *et al.* 1997), play down the significance of illness (Pound *et al.* 1998), redefine the meaning of health (Charles and Walters 1998) or claim moral validity from the way they strive to control (Adams *et al.* 1997) or fight the illness (Pollock 1995). Private accounts, by contrast, 'refer to meanings derived from the ... world of body experience and pain ... including all those difficult and socially unacceptable aspects of body experience and outpourings like blood, vomit and faeces' (Kelly and Field 1996: 250).

Decisions to ask for medical advice are further influenced by socially constructed beliefs about whether the condition is amenable to treatment and by the stigma associated with illness. Internalised assumptions about the inevitability of ill health in old age – as well as self-reliance – may explain why Charles and Walters (1998) found that many older women who knew they had arthritis were reluctant to consult their doctors. Older people from minority ethnic groups in

Liverpool also described a variety of socially constructed barriers to seeking medical help (Boneham *et al.* 1997: 178):

- internalised ageism: 'There is nothing the doctor can do. It is just old age';
- fear of professional intervention: 'He is frightened of going in a home';
- resistance to medical treatment: 'I don't believe in tablets'; and
- previous experience of racism: 'Wherever we go we are criticised because we are black'.

Access to NHS services

When lay people decide to consult a doctor or other health professional, they can face practical, inter-personal and emotional obstacles. Making appointments and attending surgery are influenced by material and social factors such as access to a telephone, the availability of accessible transport, the possibility and consequences of taking time off work, and caring responsibilities (Cornwell 1984; Graham 1993). Access may also depend upon overcoming prejudicial attitudes in health professionals which are feared by, and found by, gay men (Taylor and Robertson 1994), lesbian women (Wilton 1998), disabled people (Oliver 1990), older people (Sidell 1995), women in general (Foster 1995; Gannon 1998) and Black people (Ahmad 1993).

Women have higher rates of GP consultation than men, but research by Popay *et al.* (1993) and Wyke *et al.* (1998) suggests that both women and men are equally likely to consult their GP for similar symptoms and that women's greater levels of attendance reflect real physical and psychological differences. Smaje and Le Grand (1997) found that certain minority ethnic groups (the Chinese population, young Pakistani women and African Caribbean men) show a low use of GP services compared to the majority population, but again that raised rates of GP consultation by other minority ethnic groups mainly reflect higher levels of sickness.

While there is almost universal use of GPs, equality of access is a complex issue (Carr-Hill *et al.* 1996; Worrall *et al.* 1997). A variety of factors affects access to health and social services, for sufferers and carers alike. These include covert discrimination on grounds of age (Henwood 1991; O'Neill 1996), associated with sexual orientation (Aronson 1998), or due to racial identity (Ahmad 1993). Institutionalised discrimination is also widely seen in such areas as:

- the inequitable geographical distribution of NHS services, for example between inner-city and suburban districts (Curtis and Rees Jones 1998);
- the failure to match service users' first language (Ahmad and Walker 1997); and
- differential knowledge about services and rights, for example between different ethnic groups (Atkin and Rollings 1993; Ahmad and Atkin 1996; Ahmad and Walker 1997).

Unequal treatment is additionally evident in how patients are dealt with by medical staff and in the likelihood of referral beyond the GP, reflecting wider inequalities in power in the relationship between patients, their families and GPs (and other health and social care professionals). Less well-educated patients are likely to be given shorter consultations and poorer patients are less likely to be referred for specialist opinion or to be offered an operation (Worrall *et al.* 1997). There is evidence of reduced levels of referral of members of minority ethnic groups to in-patient and (especially) out-patient services (Cooper *et al.* 1998b; Smaje and Le Grand 1997), and of relatively low-risk, white, male, middle-aged heart-attack survivors having priority for NHS rehabilitation services and by-pass surgery (Petticrew *et al.* 1993).

Where professionals do not take lay health workers seriously, perhaps because of judgements based on social status (Roberts 1985), delays in identifying life-threatening illness can result. Sloper (1996) found wide variations in length of time before diagnosis following an initial consultation with a GP for symptoms relating to childhood cancer. A common theme was that parents felt they had not been listened to: "'Nobody believed he was ill. Everyone was saying it was psychological. I didn't think it was. People were trying to say it was because I was a single parent'" (Sloper 1996: 193).

Outside the NHS, access to both private and commercial treatment and care is unequally distributed because these depend upon the ability to pay. Private health care is widely used, with over-the-counter medication substantially exceeding the volume of prescribed drugs (Stacey 1988). Aids and adaptations, special clothing, health foods, special diets and alternative or complementary medical treatments are commonly and increasingly purchased (Sharma 1992).

Once treatment is prescribed, active participation by patients and carers in following treatment regimes is required. Goldstein and Rivers (1996) found that a large proportion of carers of older people took some responsibility for medication. This included ordering and collecting repeat prescriptions, collecting medication from the chemist, administering treatments, opening child-proof containers and monitoring and prompting medication management. Parents of children with cystic fibrosis are relied on by professionals to maintain a regime of physiotherapy, diet and medication (Eiser *et al.* 1995). The toll on the parents, the child and their siblings – and on their relationships with each other – that results from the stress of keeping to this discipline even when the child is well is very apparent. In such circumstances the significance of unequally distributed material and social resources for the quality of life of those living with ill health is considerable.

The distribution of social and material resources

When living with ill health, people value many kinds of resource, not simply professional health care, as contributing to improved quality of life. Here we will focus on two: material resources and supportive social relationships. In each case the experience of illness is permeated by socially created inequalities, for, as Giddens argues, 'Resources are ... the media through which power is exercised routinely in social interaction and through which structures of domination are reproduced' (cited in Thorogood 1989: 321).

Material resources

A consistent theme in accounts of the experience of profound ill health is the significance of material resources for quality of life. First, illness brings unavoidable additional costs associated with care and treatment (such as heating, equipment or transport). For example, around a third of people with cancer surveyed by MORI in 1992 for the Cancer Relief MacMillan Fund – and a larger proportion of carers – said they had spent significantly more money on petrol and heating since diagnosis.

Second, extra expenditure may alleviate to some degree the destructive effects of serious and long-term illness. Beresford *et al.* (1996: 39) describe this as the development of 'different priorities, especially when a child is ill, in pain, in hospital or simply needs to be stimulated or entertained'. Outings, holidays and celebrations positively affect the struggle to manage illness and reduce the negative consequences of ill health. On the other hand, the experience of illness is associated with additional disabling barriers to such activities, including difficulties in securing travel insurance or in accessing public buildings.

Third, under current social conditions, illness threatens both short- and long-term income and financial security (Ahmad and Atkin 1996). The likelihood of having financial reserves, health insurance or flexible working conditions which allow for the management of fluctuating health is related to occupation and employment. Yet those most likely to experience ill health are least likely to have these occupational advantages. This operates in a variety of complex ways. For example, accounts of chronic obstructive airways disease (COAD) showed that the greater personal control over the work process experienced by non-manual as compared with manual workers offered the chance of continuing in work far longer (Williams 1993). For families where a child had contracted cancer, Sloper's (1996) research demonstrated gender differences in the impact on employment: 50 per cent of mothers and 37 per cent of fathers who were previously in work were negatively affected. Mothers commonly lost work, reduced hours and responsibilities or took sick-leave, while fathers suffered in terms of stress and tiredness, difficulties in keeping up with work and not being allowed enough time off. Twice as many fathers as mothers commented positively on the effects of support from employers. The combination of employment costs and financial difficulties were reflected in significantly higher 'malaise' scores for parents whose work was negatively affected or who were not in work.

The experience of ill health in the absence of adequate material resources can constitute a major threat to self-esteem. One study of the value of preventive services revealed the particular importance to older women of their home's appearance:

> The ... appearance of the home could impact upon older people's comfort, sense of well-being and social participation ... The public identities of older people, and in particular women, were very tied up with the presentation of their homes to the outside world. Their home became a demonstration of their competence as adult members of the community and therefore its appearance was an important factor in feeling included in society ... Keeping the house up was akin to keeping themselves up.
>
> (Joseph Rowntree Foundation 1998c: 2)

Such threats to personal identity are much reduced where people have the resources to purchase help, maintain their home's physical condition and support reciprocal relationships (Qureshi and Walker 1989).

Moreover for many people, living with ill health is compounded by constant worries over lack of money. Ahmad and Walker (1997) reported that 32 per cent of their Bradford sample of Asian older people who were facing ill health worried much of the time about being able to pay for food, and large percentages were anxious about paying other bills and about meeting family obligations.

Supportive social relationships: Social capital

Supportive social relationships are a second major resource affecting quality of life in ill health. Social relationships generally, not just informal care, are protective of both quality and length of life but are unequally patterned by social factors (Means 1997). Bowling *et al.* (1997) found that men over 85 with few social ties had a higher risk of death during a follow-up period of thirty months, while being active in social clubs seemed protective of women's survival; over time, 'losses in number of friends was associated with worsening life satisfaction' (Joseph Rowntree Foundation 1997: 2). Older people living in the inner city were less likely to have retained close friendships or to have strong family ties.

This was echoed in Richardson and Pearson's (1995) study of thirty-seven inner-city respondents who had been assessed as needing either district nursing, home care or both. Loneliness, bereavement and isolation were the most significant problems identified, particularly by those respondents with long-term health problems who lived alone (59 per cent of the sample). Several participants appeared to be suffering from severe or prolonged grief: "'I've got no near relatives. I might as well be alone in the world ... Monday, I sat in that chair over there and I sobbed my heart out"' (Richardson and Pearson 1995: 282). When asked what kind of help they would value the majority said they would like to go out more. But, particularly for those who as a result of disablist barriers, poverty and feeling unwell had become resigned to not going out, the absence of close personal contact was the primary concern. Sloper (1996) also reported that parents of a child with cancer who felt they had no one to talk to outside the immediate family were significantly more likely to have high malaise scores. Relatives and friends were most likely to be mentioned as valuable in this respect, ahead of spouses or professionals.

The availability of informal care resources is significantly influenced by gender differences. Inequalities are particularly acute in extreme old age, when women are very much less likely than men to have a spouse or partner living in the household with them and hence are much more likely to have to rely on external informal or formal resources (Bywaters and Harris 1998). There are other significant ways in which the resource of informal care is influenced by social inequalities. For example, the availability of extended family support amongst Asian communities is curtailed as a consequence of economic and social policies, affecting immigration, employment and housing patterns (Butt and Mirza 1996). Older lesbians and gay men may also have attenuated social relationships because of rejection by their families (Aronson 1998; Bayliss forthcoming).

Moreover, many social work service users will have less substantial social networks than does the population as a whole. For example, opportunities to develop and maintain social relations are affected by factors such as financial costs and discrimination (Qureshi and Walker 1989). People with learning disabilities may have been actively discouraged from getting married or forming lifelong partnerships and may have had restricted opportunities for developing social relationships because of the attitudes of formal and informal caregivers (Williams 1992).

SOCIAL WORK ENGAGEMENT 1: COMPOUNDING INEQUALITIES

These illustrations of the permeation of ill health by social inequalities have not included one important dimension: the availability of formal support services provided through professional social workers. In discussing this aspect, the focus will mainly be on the statutory roles and responsibilities of local authority social services departments for community care, although parallels can be drawn for childcare policy and practice (Bywaters 1996). We examine, first, the consequences of key features of community care policy for inequalities in health and, second, evidence about social work practice within that framework.

Neither mainstream social workers/care managers nor social services departments are responsible for the policy framework within which they have to operate. Blackman and Atkinson (1997) describe the combination of substantial unmet need, published eligibility crit-eria and insufficient cash-limited budgets as putting care managers in an impossible position. As Tanner (1998: 453) vividly expresses it: 'Practitioners are required to behave in a disempowering way but to believe that they are in the business of empowering those who are oppressed.' However, this does not mean that the negative consequences of current practice for inequalities in health can be ignored. We begin the examination of how social services can compound health inequalities by looking briefly at three key features of the social policy framework: inadequate resources, targeting, and the relationship between formal services and informal carers.

Inequalities in the policy framework

Inadequate resources, inadequate services

As Means and Smith (1998) observe, the complexity of the funding system for community care makes any clear judgement about the adequacy of funding difficult. However, while it is widely accepted that spending on the NHS requires above-inflation increases to keep pace with demand and new treatments, the base budget for local authority social services has been progressively cut. Edwards and Kenny (1997) state that Government support for social services fell 6 per cent in the previous five years. In 1996–7, sixty-nine of the 119 English local authorities made service cuts of £166 m., efficiency savings of £69m. and increased anticipated revenues from charges by £27m. compared to the previous year (Means and Smith 1998). The largest cuts made during this period were in services for older people, reflected in a drop both in the number of older people in residential care, from 314,500 in 1992 to 297,400 in 1998, and in the numbers being provided with care at home through local authorities, down from 529,000 in 1992 to 471,000 in 1997 (Inman 1999). As demonstrated throughout this book, this pattern of reductions in both expenditure on and the provision of social care has taken place against a background of increasing need.

Despite the public commitment of the Labour Government to increase expenditure over the period 1999–2002, Chris Davies, president of the ADSS, argued at a national conference in January 1999 that the targets set could only be achieved under three conditions:

- if there was a realistic annual uprating of base budgets (which had not been seen in the 1998–9 settlement);
- if further policy initiatives, such as the Carers Strategy to be announced in 1999, were accompanied by additional money; and
- if there was a recognition that local authorities were starting from the position of being unable to meet existing required standards.

As social workers working as care managers are only too aware (Tanner 1998), inadequate resources mean inadequate service provision for people who consequently face unnecessary suffering. To take one example, for some this means that basic expectations associated with self-esteem and identity, such as the right to be clean (Ottewill *et al.* 1996), are in doubt. Richardson and Pearson (1995) found high levels of unmet need for assistance with bathing which had been exacerbated by health and safety legislation. Means (1997: 416) reported the example of a respondent who 'had been told she could not have help to have a bath in her home and so the only option was to have a bath in a residential home which would involve an expensive taxi journey'. What this represents is socially created inequalities in the experience of ill health.

Inequalities exacerbated by targeting

The strategy of targeting community care services, through the application of eligibility criteria coupled with means tests, stands in contrast with current policies for the NHS, which still largely provides services free at the point of delivery. This produces inequalities in two main ways. First, as Blackman and Atkinson (1997) suggest, the system is inequitable because it relies on expressed or referred needs which, in turn, depend on knowledge of services and willingness to refer. Yet Ahmad and Walker found that only 60 per cent of elderly respondents from Asian minority groups in Bradford had heard of social workers, while knowledge of other community care services was below 50 per cent. Women were particular poorly informed: 'Relatively few know about available services; fewer still use them. The onus on providing interpreters remains with the users themselves' (Ahmad and Walker 1997: 161). Moreover, as we discuss below, maintaining self-esteem may require that poor health is played down, while the perceived family orientation of social services may deter those, such as older lesbians (Bayliss forthcoming), who anticipate that their needs will not be met.

Second, when the strategy of targeting is combined with inadequate resources it inevitably leads to a situation in which 'only those at the highest dependency end ... will get any kind of service at all' and 'preventive services risk being seen as a luxury' (Means 1997: 410). As a result, services become increasingly concentrated. Indeed, Blackman and Atkinson (1997) report a fall of 5 per cent in the number of households receiving local authority home-care services between 1994 and 1995, while the range of tasks undertaken has also been reduced (Richardson and Pearson 1995; Blackman and Atkinson 1997), excluding much work vital to self-esteem and social participation.

This raises the prospect of a growing social care divide. The better-off will meet their multiple 'low-level' needs through paying for care, while others may be forced to wait until a crisis propels them into the high-need categories which generate a response from social services (Means 1997).

Inequalities in support for informal carers

'Caring for People' recognised explicitly that 'the great bulk of community care is provided by friends, family and neighbours' (DoH 1989: 4). The dependence on women was not acknowledged. Eleven years later a Social Services Inspectorate (SSI) inquiry into local authority support for carers (Fruin 1998) focused on inequalities within and between local authorities, according to location, client group and between ethnic minority and majority populations, but still made no mention of gender inequalities in the giving and receiving of informal care. There remains little sign of any significant move towards the structural changes required to make decisions to provide care and to receive informal care into matters of genuine choice (Morris 1993). Moreover, there is some evidence to suggest that, despite awareness amongst care managers of the gender inequalities of caring, services may still be more likely to provide support to male than to female carers in situations of equal need (Bywaters and Harris 1998).

That inequalities in informal care are compounded by social services policy and practice is apparent in Blackman and Atkinson's

(1997) comparison of two groups of people aged over 75. The formal and informal support available to one group who had been assessed for social services was compared with that obtainable by another group living in similar financial circumstances. In both groups informal care proved to be a substitute for formal care, an almost inevitable consequence in a situation of scarce resources in the absence of explicit local authority policies about eligibility, and was being inadequately supported. Of the group assessed for social services, 33 per cent said there was help that they needed but were not getting, but when they were living with others this rose to 57 per cent. The widespread failure to inform carers of their entitlement to an assessment, to make such an assessment and to involve carers in decisions about services provided, reported by Fruin (1998), can only compound these institutionalised, gendered inequalities.

The general charge that social services' policy compounds health inequalities is also reflected in a number of respects in the specifics of practice to which we now turn.

Inequalities in practice

A lack of awareness of the significance of illness in service users' lives

Several studies point to a lack of awareness amongst social workers of the significance of ill health in service users' lives. This is reflected in Corney's (1985) study of a generic intake team (albeit now rather dated and containing problematic and potentially overlapping categories) which showed that less than 10 per cent of the subjects of referrals where the identified 'client' was over 16 were in good physical health. Almost two-thirds (of 117) described themselves as suffering from a 'chronic illness' or a 'major disability'. In addition, eight service users were not included in the study because they had been admitted to hospital and two had died. Another 25 per cent described themselves as having 'one or more *minor* symptoms such as frequent headaches, leg pains, stomach pains etc.' (Corney 1985: 874, our emphasis).

However, as shown in Table 4:1, social workers were found to underestimate substantially the extent and significance of this ill health in their service users' lives. Around 40 per cent of users who described themselves as living with a 'chronic illness' or 'major

Table 4.1 Reported ill health and social workers' assessments

Service users' self-reported ill health (percentages)		Social workers' assessements of service users' ill health		
		None	Minor	Major
None or symptomatic	41	39	2	0
Chronic illness	29	15	6	8
Major disability	47	15	21	11

Source: Corney (1985)

disability' were assessed by the social workers as having no health problems, while 'minor' symptoms went almost unnoticed.

Evidence of social workers' failure to pick up and act on the physical health-related needs of service users is underlined by two other sources. Howells' (1986) article on medical needs of 'mentally handicapped' adults revealed 203 unmanaged physical health conditions amongst a group of 151 people attending a 'training centre'. Redmond *et al.* (1996) investigated untreated health problems in seventy-seven older people receiving home care. Sixty-eight were assessed as likely to benefit from further intervention from health care services; in total 192 referrals were made, including thirty-six to GPs. Levels of unmet health need were significantly higher in the group receiving home care than in a control group who were not in contact with social services.

The health needs of children looked after by social services authorities have recently become a target for attention (DoH 1998d) following evidence which revealed a similar failure to record or even to identify their health status (Bywaters 1996). 'Achieving or maintaining a reasonable standard of health' is, of course, a key part of the legal definition of children in need (The Children Act S17: 10). However, the authors have been unable to locate any recent UK studies explicitly detailing the extent of ill health amongst children and young people in contact with social services but not 'looked after', despite their being at high risk of the illnesses, accidents and impairments associated with relative poverty and disadvantaged environmental circumstances.

The narrow scope of assessment

The experience and meaning of illness reflected in outline earlier in this chapter cannot be captured by assessment processes which consider health in terms of formulaic representations of 'activities of daily living' or which ignore interactions between poverty and poor health. As Lewis and Glennerster (1996) imply, the focus on determining priorities for service provision has meant that physical illness has become a trigger for establishing eligibility, rather than an indication of possible further needs to be explored and met, primary problems to be resolved or mitigated, or preventive action to be undertaken. A degree of recovery from illness, by removing users from the highest risk category, could mean the removal of the very services which were underpinning that improvement.

Moreover, as Tanner (1998: 451) argues, service users are disempowered by stigmatising assessment processes which not only focus on what service users and carers cannot manage (rather than what they can) but require practitioners to 'stress the magnitude of their problems in order to demonstrate their eligibility'. In contrast with this perverse incentive to emphasise 'incapacity', Cornwell's (1984) experience of talking to working-class people in east London about their health was that accounts given to officials emphasised the 'morally correct' position of being basically healthy. As Annandale (1998: 27) puts it: 'The quest to be seen as "healthy" bore no necessary relation to an individual's medical history. Indeed, Cornwell recounts instances where her respondents described a series of quite serious health problems but still described themselves as "healthy".' This assertion of being 'well' was part of a process of maintaining a public reputation and self-esteem which, as we have seen earlier, is in itself important for health. Poverty also carries stigma, so securing a full assessment of the twin effects of poverty and poor health is necessarily a skilful process. Forms of practice 'dominated by unimaginative, routinized, bureaucratic approaches' (Lymbery 1998: 875) are unlikely to facilitate this.

Professional social work has made significant changes over the last twenty years in its commitment to anti-oppressive practice in assessment, but this is not necessarily reflected in practice. When service users' ethnic identity is ignored or marginalised or when the assessment of carers' needs is a matter of chance (Fruin 1998), this is rightly a focus of attention. There has been no parallel concern about inequalities in ill health.

The narrow range of provision

The current policy and resource framework for community care, a lack of awareness of physical health and a narrow focus of assessment combine to result in limited service provision which does not meet those needs associated with illness outlined earlier. A number of studies have pointed up the reduction in the range of services provided in many authorities, with some withdrawing from aspects of provision such as household cleaning (Blackman and Atkinson 1997; Means 1997; Richardson and Pearson 1995). As a result the SSI report on home care services (1998b) gives evidence of wide geographical inequalities, with service users in some areas having little chance of having their house or windows cleaned or meals prepared (Table 4:2). Further differences in service provision according to gender, ethnic identity or health status may have been present, but no evidence of these was presented.

Richardson and Pearson (1995: 284) found that 'highly constrained resources' led to home care services designed to support 'minimal physical maintenance based on a model of dependency, rather than ... to maximise their independence by preventive or rehabilitative social care'. This meant that respondents were 'clearly upset that ... they were unable to maintain their personal standards or social roles as they would have wished'. For example, in relation to help with shopping, 'home helps' did not usually have enough time to go the main shopping centres (where prices would be cheaper), to take service users with them when shopping (with associated social, physical and emotional benefits) or to enable users to exercise choice, for example over the selection of presents or clothes. Recognition of the inadequacy of what they were allowed to offer in worktime was shown by home helps' provision of additional services in their own time.

Table 4.2 Variation in service provision across nine local authorities

Service	Proportion of users receiving help
House cleaning	26–86%
Preparing meals	16–52%
Window cleaning	0–41%
Washing/bathing	27–94%
Help during the night	2–26%

Source: Social Services Inspectorate 1998b

Despite the evidence of emotional suffering accompanying ill health presented earlier, the SSI (1998b) inspection of home care also demonstrates the relatively limited priority given to 'social and emotional support' by statutory providers. This was received by only 33 per cent of those using home care services. Support for 'socialising', 'leisure, recreation', 'religious and cultural activities', 'community links' or 'neighbourhood activities' averaged less than 10 per cent across all nine authorities despite the evidence of the value of social support in managing illness.

Other studies report a number of further major consequences of care managers' limited conception of their role in relation to illness. These include a lack of recognition of people's need for information about their illness and about services and resources they may value (Ahmad and Atkin 1996; Beresford *et al.* 1996; Joseph Rowntree *Findings* 1998a); not taking the role of health advocacy (Dunning 1995) or assisting in the management of medication and treatment (Goldstein and Rivers 1996); and failing to assist service users and carers to become engaged with self-help initiatives (Simpson 1996).

Unmet need

Recording unmet need is one way in which social workers could give recognition to the conditions service users faced despite the resource and policy constraints curtailing current practice. Local authorities have been reluctant to record unmet need (Blackman and Atkinson 1997), but this has not been effectively challenged by practitioners or the professional organisations. As Drakeford (1998: 225) argues, 'budget inadequacies and cut-backs have been too easily accommodated into practice in a way which justifies and defends rationing, rather than protesting and campaigning against the effects upon individuals who have no recourse to funds of their own.' This reflects a wider failure to engage with an 'epidemiological' (population-wide) approach to social care needs which would demonstrate links between social inequalities and service provision.

SOCIAL WORK ENGAGEMENT 2: TOWARDS MORE EQUALISING PRACTICE

Notwithstanding social work's complicity in policies and practices which perpetuate rather than reduce inequalities in the course of ill health, it does have a more positive contribution to make. Three main conclusions can be drawn from the evidence presented so far. First, as is apparent throughout, greater equality in the experience of ill health depends fundamentally on the redistribution of economic, environmental and social resources within the population as a whole and, as a secondary measure, on enhanced funding for health and social services.

Second, to maximise its impact on health inequalities, social work has to move beyond the constraints exemplified in the dominant forms of contemporary social services departmental structures, policies and practices. This involves greater awareness by social workers within, as well as beyond, social services departments of the extent and significance of illness in the lives of service users and the non-stigmatising provision of an appropriate range of services which allow people to maximise their health potential and minimise unnecessary suffering. Social workers should focus on supporting service users' own agendas in managing their ill health. They should also recognise the impact of ill health on other aspects of service users' lives – and neither reduce concern with ill health to the question of whether or not it simply triggers service eligibility, nor assume that the resolution of health care problems is the exclusive domain of the medical and allied professions.

Third, the experience of ill health from the perspective of the people immediately concerned and their supporters shows that there is substantial scope for social work involvement. This encompasses action to:

- secure greater equality of access to existing health and social services;
- shift the balance of power in negotiating treatment and care away from health and social work professionals towards lay health workers; and
- equalise the material and social resources necessary to recovery or, in the case of continuing ill health, to enhance the quality of life.

These three dimensions of practice are now discussed, drawing on selected examples from statutory sector, voluntary sector and self-help activity.

Greater equality of access to existing services

Wider access to existing services can be secured both by providing services in settings which create ease of access on a non-stigmatising basis and by focusing on populations rather than on individuals. The main evidence for this comes from the impact of placing social services department workers in primary health care (PHC) settings. This has been found to enhance access in a number of key respects.

First, as Cumella *et al.* (undated) state, evidence that PHC-based social work *increases access* to social services provision is long established. In the four recent studies carried out by Cumella and colleagues (Cumella 1994; Cumella *et al.* undated; Grattan *et al.* 1995; Le Mesurier and Cumella 1996) and confirmed by Ross and Tissier (1997), PHC-attached social workers dealt with substantially more referrals than colleagues in community-based social services teams. In South Worcestershire there were 75 per cent more referrals to PHC-attached social workers per head of population served, including more 'high priority' cases (Cumella *et al.* undated).

Second, these additional referrals were primarily referrals by GPs of service users who *would not otherwise have accessed* needed services. As almost 100 per cent of the population is registered with a GP but significant proportions are ill informed about, unaware or suspicious of social services, using primary care as a point of referral has considerable potential for offering enhanced access.

Third, the PHC base means that, as service users emphasised to Claridge and Rivers (1997: 38), there is '*no stigma* attached to being referred to a named social worker'. Service users were also more satisfied with the service, including (another widely reported finding) the speed of initial response.

Fourth, across the studies, PHC-attached social workers took on a *wider mix of referrals*, including lower eligibility cases. This suggests that practice-based workers were able to tackle the lower level needs – the preventive agenda – which have otherwise been widespread victims of cuts in service provision. Moreover in South Worcestershire, subject of the largest study (Cumella *et al.* undated), the fewer and shorter stays in hospital which characterised service users of PHC-attached workers, reflected in the way these workers supported their service users through the process of hospitalisation and in arranging discharge, were perhaps evidence of the value of early intervention. They also appeared to result in significant reductions in care costs.

Finally, whereas referrals by GPs to area teams focused primarily on the provision of routinised practical service provision, referrals to PHC-attached workers included those requiring the *full assessment of the physical, emotional and social demands associated with severe health problems* faced by individuals. GPs in all studies valued the contact with social workers, commenting particularly on the value of feedback about the outcome of referrals made.

In addition to these positive consequences of identifying PHC as a key point for equalising and increasing access to social services for individuals, access can be enhanced through taking a population-wide approach. For example, the multi-fund Primary Care Group pilot project in Kingston and Richmond upon Thames was established partly out of ethical objections to GP fundholding and a commitment to the principles of equal access to treatment. A strategy was adopted which took a pro-active approach involving preventive interventions targeted on populations at relative risk of neglect of their health care requirements, and reviews of service provision to disadvantaged groups. One specific example was a review of access to services for people with learning disabilities (Dinsdale 1998).

An alternative population-based model for increasing non-stigmatising access is demonstrated in the Barnardos' Sherwood Project[3] for individuals with cystic fibrosis and their families. Cystic fibrosis (CF) is an inherited condition characterised by long-term digestive and respiratory symptoms. A carefully controlled and supplemented diet together with a demanding physiotherapy regime to aid breathing and help clear lung congestion are required to maximise health and life expectancy. Significant proportions of the population of the UK are carriers of the genes which can lead to a child being born with the condition; about one in twenty-five white British adults are carriers of the trait (Anionwu 1993). The families of all new-born babies diagnosed with CF in the locality of the Sherwood Project – or when a diagnosis is established later in childhood – are routinely referred to the Project regardless of individual circumstances or the severity of the condition. This universal approach to access obviates both stigma and inequalities resulting from reliance on individual lay and professional workers' knowledge of services.

Shifting the balance of power

Ill health threatens people's control over their lives, not primarily because of its physical impact but because of its social accompaniments, including the need to negotiate treatment and care with health and social care professionals in a situation of unequal power. This is particularly the case when ill health is accompanied by other dimensions of disadvantage such as poverty, or when the social relations of health care are permeated by discriminatory attitudes or institutionalised practices such as ageist or racist assumptions. Social work practice can act in a number of ways to support lay health workers in their efforts to equalise these power relations.

Information

As AIDS treatment activists were especially acute in recognising (Watney 1996), information – being informed – is particularly important to the dynamics of negotiations with professionals, as well as to the direct work of managing ill health. This is also reflected in the approach of the Sherwood Project. Throughout, people with CF and their families are offered information about the impact of CF and its treatments through 'new diagnosis groups' and educational groups focusing on particularly stressful aspects of managing the condition, such as eating strategies or the physiotherapy regime which is taught to parents. Children, as well as parents, are helped to make informed choices about treatment options.

The significance of – and the deficit in meeting – information needs is widely reflected in the work of self-help groups. For example, Cancerlink[4] runs a telephone information service about cancer, cancer treatments and cancer care. It has also provided support to about 300 local cancer self-help groups throughout the UK. It publishes a range of educational materials to underpin the effective setting up and running of local groups, and provides start-up grants, courses, workshops and conferences. Cancerlink has run action research projects to enhance the opportunities for members of minority ethnic groups to access such resources. This work exemplifies the fact that information is required not only about the condition itself but about the variety of circumstances which impact on managing ill health, including the full range of mainstream services and alternative provisions.

Towards lay control

In addition to facilitating service users' access and helping them gain information, social workers can act to equalise power relations concerning the control of treatment and care, by supporting lay activism at an individual and collective level.

Employing health advocacy to break racist barriers to accessing treatment is exemplified in locality-based work with members of the Yemeni community. Profiling the population of the Sparkbrook and

Sparkhill wards in Birmingham as part of the locality management approach revealed not only a general difficulty in accessing health information and services for members of ethnic minority communities, but also that small communities within the area – such as the Yemeni community – were particularly poorly served by all the mainstream services (Weaver 1996). With Yemeni representative involvement on the steering committee from the start, a health advoc-acy project worker was appointed, initially for a three-year period. She adopted a community development approach, beginning by building networks of contacts, particularly with women, through existing and newly developed Yemeni groups. Responding to the expressed needs encountered, she provided information on a variety of issues, including women's health and hospital and clinic appointment systems. She acted as an advocate, both on an individual and on a community basis. She accompanied individuals to contacts with a range of appointments, concerned not only with health services but also with material resources such as housing and benefits. In addition she worked to raise awareness of Yemeni culture among a range of professionals. A variety of materials was produced in English and in Arabic (both written and pictorial) as a resource for community members and professionals alike. Subsequently at the request of the community, specific events were targeted at men and families, to supplement the work already under way with women. Lessons from the project have been embedded in mainstream service delivery (locality resource manager, personal communication 1999).

At the Sherwood Project, too, social workers have highlighted, challenged and changed some patterns of treatment prescribed by consultants that have had an unnecessarily detrimental effect on the lives of CF sufferers, such as those involving long or frequent hospital stays which could disrupt schooling and lead to social isolation.

The collective basis of self-help activity that targets social disadvantage underwrites further possibilities for challenging or changing professional service provision (Evans 1996). On a neighbourhood basis, PHC-attached social workers were involved in servicing a self-help health care initiative in Northern Ireland that took the form of regular meetings of patient groups. Patients evaluated the sessions as contributing to a significant growth in self-confidence that resulted in reduced levels of medication. A further outcome of the work was that the patients concerned produced educational materials for use with other patients, including the preparation of a video (McCann and Wisener 1989/90).

On a national and international basis, self-organisation of people with ME (chronic fatigue syndrome or post-viral fatigue syndrome) through the ME movement has been at the forefront of the fight to secure recognition of the condition by the medical profession as a physical reality rather than as a purely psychological phenomenon. They have begun to make headway on this, with multiple consequences in terms of rights – in employment, to benefits and services and in reducing the stigma of accusations of malingering (Hume *et al.* 1998). Moreover, resources have been acquired for further research and influence has been exerted on the medical profession itself to support their position. The final act of the retiring chief medical officer, Kenneth Calnan, in 1998 was to announce the establishment of a DoH working group on the clinical management of ME/CFS, acknowledging that it is 'a real medical condition with debilitating and distressing results' (Hume *et al.* 1998: 3). To avoid incorporation, the ME Association is seeking direct representation and monitoring the remit of the group and its objectives.

A rights-based approach

Increasingly, self-help groups are adopting a rights-based approach to the experience of ill health, overturning the traditional expert–patient model. For example, representatives of local cancer self-help groups across the country have drawn up a 'Declaration of Rights' of people with cancer (Cancerlink undated). This reflects the agenda of shifting the balance of power between professionals and service users in a number of significant respects:

• The adoption of a rights-based approach addressed to 'health professionals, employers and the public at large' underscores the emphasis throughout this chapter on illness as a primary site of discrimination.
• The Declaration emphasises the importance of equality: 'I have the right to equal concern and attention whatever my gender, race, class, culture, religious belief, age, sexuality, lifestyle or degree of able-bodiedness.' Cancerlink recognises the additional discrimination which people from Black and ethnic minority communities and other groups such as lesbians may face through 'specialist' sub-networks.
• A number of statements directly address the hierarchical relations between people living with cancer, their families and professionals. They emphasise the right to sensitively-provided information, informed participation in decision-making, informed consent to

treatment and to entry in clinical trials and the right to refuse treatment or to use complementary therapies without prejudice.

Equalising material and social resources

Material resources

The Cancerlink Declaration also emphasises the rights of people with cancer to adequate material and social resources to sustain them during their ill health and often painful and debilitating treatment. Social workers can contribute to securing such material and social resources, including directly provided social work and social care services. For example, in the PHC setting, the improvements in *access* discussed above have been complemented by the *provision* of a wider range of services to meet the needs of those who are living with ill health in deprived circumstances. In the PHC studies we have been discussing, as in others (Paris and Player 1993; Claridge and Rivers 1997), a repeated theme was the value placed by service users and health colleagues on the availability of financial and other kinds of advice. Benefits take-up initiatives sited in primary care settings have also been found to significantly enhance users' material resources. Paris and Player (1993) report on the placing of Citizens' Advice Bureau advice workers in primary care settings in Birmingham. Of 150 people who consulted the service over three months, 39 per cent came for financial advice, usually associated with illness. Over £58,000 owed was subsequently received, of which almost £55,000 would be recurring benefits. There was evidence that these referrals would not have been achieved by conventional services. A similar project demonstrated equivalent take-up of additional benefits and also revealed that, compared to people accessing high-street CABs, a greater proportion were aged over sixty, disabled or in poor health (Veitch 1995).

Complementing take-up programmes aimed at individuals, such as these, a number of examples exist of work to put poverty on the collective agenda of professionals in PHC settings (Blackburn 1996). Bond (1999) reports such a project using Blackburn's team training handbook. Despite organisation obstacles, team members 'enhanced their understandings of the health implications of structural factors, including income distribution and unemployment, and took steps to enable poor families ... to maximise their entitlements to welfare benefits' (Bond 1999:15).

The consequences of poor environmental conditions and poverty are highly significant for the progression of cystic fibrosis – and hence to life expectancy – through their impact on respiratory infections and diet. As a result, a major aim of the Sherwood Project is to enhance the material resources of families and young adults with CF. The Project does not simply provide information about benefits but undertakes advocacy work, which can be invaluable in supporting young adults moving out of the parental home and facing institutionalised discrimination in areas such as employment and the benefits system. It is also of crucial importance to parents themselves in continuing to hold down employment. For example, if a claim for disability living allowance is being made when the person is relatively well the chances of success are lessened, removing their entitlement when they become more severely ill. If an adult with CF – or caring for a child with CF – is in employment, taking time off when ill and attending hospital appointments when healthy can be equally problematic.

Social resources

The core activity promoted by Cancerlink is mutually supportive local group work, in which giving and receiving various forms of social support – practical, physical and emotional – are undertaken by group members and volunteers (Cancerlink 1989). A key problem that has to be negotiated is that of disablist barriers to accessing engagement in group activity in the course of profound ill health. Tele(phone)conferencing is still a relatively new phenomenon in social work in Britain (Rosenfield and Smillie 1998). Nevertheless, drawing on the input of Community Network, a charity which provides telephone conferencing facilities for other charities, Cancerlink has pioneered the use of teleconferencing in Britain as a medium for self-help support group interaction (Rosenfield and Urben 1994). At first sight teleconferencing may seem impersonal. However, evaluations indicate that it provides a vital opportunity for experiencing the warmth of human contact and the benefits of group solidarity. For example, Rosenfield and Urben's evaluation of a telephone support group for women experiencing gynaecological cancer includes the following comments from participants (1994: 22): '"... lovely feeling of friendship ... reassurance. I'm not alone with my trials, tribulations and anxieties"; "... not met anyone else with ovarian cancer. Nice to hear people a couple of years on and going strong".'

As well as focusing on material resources, the Sherwood Project works to increase the social resources of people living with CF. The information and education groups mentioned above provide opportunities for mutual support, friendship and advice as well as drawing on the technical expertise of professionals such as dieticians. Such groups not only deal with the physical aspects of the condition and forms of medical treatment for it, but also with its consequences for relationships and identity. The Project's eating group works with children as well as parents, although the risk of cross-infection makes group work with children more difficult. In addition, families are offered support through bereavements, including through play work. Examples of counselling and self-help on a group basis were also featured in PHC-based practice in Northern Ireland (McCann and Wisener 1989/90) where workers ran long-term relaxation groups as well as supporting individual relaxation programmes carried out at home.

CONCLUSION

The profound, pervasive impact of social inequalities on the experience of ill health has been evident throughout this chapter. This has underscored the need for fundamental changes in social policy and the redistribution of material and social resources across society. Social work has been revealed as – in some respects – implicated in compounding this unjust situation. However, our analysis has also shown that it can and, to some extent, does play an important role in redressing inequalities in the course of ill health. Through working to widen access to services, to tilt the balance of power away from professional control and to maximise the availability of material and social resources, social work can ally itself with the thrust of lay health activism towards greater equity in ill health.

Chapter 5

Ill health and hospitalisation

INTRODUCTION

While most health care is home-based, being a hospital patient can mark a critical juncture in living with ill health. It can represent the relief of acute or chronic pain, the treatment of profound disease or the presentation of a sobering diagnosis. It may also lead to further ill health, denote the transition to increased impairment and make heavy demands on patients themselves and those close to them. The experience of hospital treatment is also characterised by inequality.

The chances of treatment and recovery for hospital patients, together with the demands they face, do not only arise from ill health in itself. For a large percentage of the hospital population, in-patient experience is permeated by the rigours of a system of care characterised by inequitable resourcing. Further dimensions to social disadvantage, such as ageism and racism, are reflected in discrimination in the course of hospitalisation. Becoming a patient also opens up the possibility of a subordinating response from health care professionals. In this chapter we examine the impact on health of inequality in the course of hospital care, how social work is enmeshed in this, but also how it can contribute to more equitable outcomes for health.

Current debates in the UK about the efficacy of hospital-related social work concentrate on its involvement in planning discharge from hospital (Davies and Connolly 1995b, Rachman 1993). We deliberately widen the discussion to incorporate, in addition to discharge planning, the following key phases of hospitalisation: care on leaving hospital, and experience as an in-patient. In each case we discuss:

- the inequitable policy backdrop to the efforts of hospital patients, social workers and health service colleagues;
- the major obstacles patients have to negotiate to obtain equitable treatment; and
- social work's current contribution to securing a more equal chance of well-being for hospital patients.

Finally, we consider how social work could contribute more effectively to greater equality in health in the course of hospitalisation.

Social work concerned with hospitalisation is commonly treated as marginal, lacking the organisational prestige of major sectors of practice such as child-care (McLeod 1995a). With few exceptions, there is also a dearth of systematic British research on its significance (Davies and Connolly 1995a). Yet as we will show, it should be viewed as a central facet of practice, with the potential to make an important contribution to greater equity in health and well-being.

Questions of definition and selectivity

While arguing for the crucial importance of hospital-based social work, we also acknowledge the relevance to patients' welfare of practice initiatives *not* based in hospital, but linked to hospitalisation. Hence our definition of hospital social work is social work concerned with the *process of hospitalisation*. We also regard an appropriate public health approach as one that does not stop at the hospital door. A process of hospitalisation that incorporates social work presents an important opportunity for promoting health and preventing unnecessary illness – for example, through maximising chances of recovery – and attention to the economic, social and environmental determinants of health is intrinsic to effective hospital care.

Dealing with such a large and intricate area of experience as being a hospital patient necessitates some selectivity, and so our account mainly focuses on older people. First, the majority of in-patients are older people. Two-thirds of admissions to the specialty of general medicine are of people aged 65 years or over (Audit Commission 1992). Second, it is important to challenge the stigmatising treatment of this group in public debate. In a cruel inversion of reality, older people's use of hospital care has been framed as problematic on the grounds that it is excessive (O'Neill 1996). On the contrary, as our account confirms, their use of hospital resources is problematic only because so frequently they receive inadequate care.

We also do not focus in the main on out-patient and day treatment because regrettably this remains such an underdeveloped site of hospital social work activity. The drive within the NHS to speed up 'patient throughput', coupled with underfunded SSDs' increasingly narrow focus on 'core business', have combined to pressurise hospital social work to concentrate increasingly on swiftly executed discharge planning (personal communication, British Association of Social Workers, Health-related Special Interest Group (BASWHRSIG) 1998). This is despite the rapid growth of out-patient and day treatments and their potential importance for preventive social work, with opportunities for early appraisal of serious problems and advance planning (Bedics 1994).

IN-PATIENT EXPERIENCE AND HOSPITAL SOCIAL WORK

In theory, social workers on site in hospital are well placed to draw attention to, or address, the social problems which undermine people's well-being as in-patients. This is all the more important in the light of recent evidence on the rigours of being an in-patient in the face of the inequities of underfunding and the persistence of entrenched hierarchies and discrimination in hospital treatment. Sadly, as we will show, hospital-based social work's engagement with the socially created problems faced by in-patients is itself bogged down by underfunding, and by discriminatory practices beyond and within social work, despite all the efforts of hospital social workers themselves.

Underfunded care: A threat to recovery

The chronic current underfunding of the NHS (see Chapter 2) is manifest in in-patients' experience. From several quarters there is worrying evidence that shortages of resources are threatening in-patients' health, representing inequitable treatment for those unable to buy themselves out of the experience of state-funded in-patient stays. Hospital-based social workers going on to wards and in contact with patients, their families and NHS staff are also in a position to be aware of the following health-damaging practices, which epitomise shortages in both staff and plant.

Going hungry

One of the most fundamental health care needs is adequate nutrition. It is of particular importance in in-patient care given that at least one in three people who have been ill for some time prior to admission will have lost weight and about one in ten will have become seriously malnourished (DoH 1995a). However, information from community health councils and an independent inquiry commissioned by the Secretary of State for Health (Health Advisory Service (HAS) 2000, 1998) provides evidence of staff being too busy – and sometimes lacking the nursing skills – to ensure that patients are adequately fed. In the process there is a disablist disregard of the requirements of physically impaired patients, with frequent accounts of meals being left and removed on the assumption that patients did not want them.

> 'The truth is if I had not visited my father at mealtimes he would not have eaten at all. I found it hard to take in but my father was left a meal and then it was collected again, with just a shout of "Not hungry again today …". The facts were that my father had very little speech and was not capable physically to move to the bottom of the bed to reach his food; even if he could have done this he was not actually able to feed himself.' (Report from Hampshire.)
> (Association of Community Health Councils
> for England and Wales (ACHCEW) 1997: 14)

ACHCEW has argued that a major reason for this problem can be found in the dramatic fall in the numbers of registered nurses on wards and deteriorating working conditions arising through additional pressures of work. Further studies endorse this point. Recruitment problems have been reported by 78 per cent of trusts (Income Data Services 1998). The Royal College of Nursing has found nurse vacancies on general medical wards are averaging 12 per cent nationally, with 95 per cent of nurses in charge of wards commenting that patient care is regularly compromised by short-staffing (White 1998).

The government has taken a series of measures to boost recruitment and retention of staff, notably the implementation of human resource management measures such as new targets for anti-harassment policies and occupational health policies (DoH 1998b), higher nurse consultant salaries (White 1998) and relatively high increases in starting salary levels (*Guardian*, 2 February 1998: 9). Nevertheless, the viewpoint of nursing organisations' leaders is that unless there is a substantial improvement in pay and conditions for all nursing staff the present shortages will continue (Payne 1998).

Unequal risk of further infection

Recent studies have shown that compounding such conditions, 10 per cent of hospital in-patients risk acquiring an infection in NHS hospitals, compared with under 1 per cent in private hospitals, specialists in hospital infection control identifying shortages in NHS funding as heavily implicated here:

> There is a strong view that hot-bedding [where the same bed is occupied by different people across a 24-hour period], the pressure on beds and the necessity for mixed-specialty wards are very difficult circumstances in which to conduct infection control.
> (Casewell quoted in the *Independent*, 29 November 1997: 7)

Further features of NHS hospital underfunding implicated in this situation are problems with keeping wards clean and in good repair which in turn reflect dilapidated building and reductions in staffing levels for cleaning (HAS 2000, 1998).

Doctor–patient hierarchies

These worrying aspects of care are accompanied by the persistence of doctor–patient hierarchies. To have patients being better informed and participating more actively in consultation is conducive to better health; patients experience less distress both during and following treatment (Rumsey and Harcourt 1998), with possibly more successful treatment outcomes (Kaplan *et al.* 1989). Increasing attention is also being paid to this in doctors' training (Soothill *et al.* 1995). Nevertheless, there continues to be evidence of routine failure to inform and consult patients about the nature and course of treatment. Tritter's (1996) study of cancer patients' views on the appropriateness of their treatment drew on twelve focus groups involving seventy-five patients with a variety of forms of cancer, across four locations. As co-workers for their own health, the patients concerned had three straightforward but key requirements (Tritter 1996: 41):

• to be given information about the disease, treatment options, side-effects and how to obtain support;

- to be able to ask, knowing that they would receive an honest answer and that they could keep on asking until they felt that their particular needs for information had been satisfied; and
- that information should be a two-way process and that health professionals needed information about their patients if they were to be effective.

In practice only one patient was completely satisfied with the amount of information they received. Many patients described feeling that doctors disapproved of them trying to obtain information or that it was being withheld (1996: 18): '"I remember when I first met my consultant he said, 'promise me darling, you'll never go to the library and look things up'" (female Hodgkins disease patient); "They were all very nice, very wonderful, but I realised afterwards that nobody told me anything" (female breast cancer patient).'
Crucial information regarding surgical procedures and outcomes was frequently lacking (1996:29).

> Very few felt that they knew what to expect from surgery. Breast cancer patients, for example, had no idea what their scar would look like after a mastectomy and were often sent home without having seen it … sometimes patients were told that the operation had been 'a success' but in very few cases was it explained what this meant.

Further discrimination

Interwoven with evidence of subordinating behaviour towards patients generally is evidence of discrimination on the basis of patients' social position. Separate studies of Kashmiri and African Caribbean patients found that serious health consequences arose from the failure of hospital treatment to meet their requirements. First, interpreters were not available when required by Kashmiri women on their own during childbirth. Moreover, it could be difficult to be certain that informed consent to an emergency caesarean section had been obtained (Imtiaz and Johnson 1993). Second, African Caribbean patients expressed disappointment at the slow progress in understanding the nature and effects of diseases 'exclusive' to themselves, reflected in insufficient pain relief being offered in frequently excruciating flare-ups of sickle cell anaemia (Johnson and Sangster 1996). Differential access to standard treatments is also well documented. For example, women are less likely than men to be offered cardiac surgery (Petticrew *et al.* 1993); older people are less likely to be offered cancer therapy (Fentiman *et al.* 1990) and kidney transplantation (O'Neill 1996).

The input of hospital-based social work

Strategically placed

Hospital-based social workers are strategically placed to combat these inequalities. First, approaching 20 per cent of SSD social workers are involved in hospital-based social work (SSI 1992a). Second, hospitals are a crucial point of access to social work services. Shaw's (1991) study of hospitals in Avon found that the majority of users of hospital social work services were not previously known to the SSD (80 per cent) but met 'greatest need criteria' involving a high probability of residential care and according to which not providing a service would put the patient or another at risk. Third, given the widespread emphasis within social work on 'anti-oppressive practice', hospital-based practice should, in theory, be alert to the ways in which social inequality permeates in-patient experience. Finally, with its long history – dating back to 1895 (Bell 1961) – what hospital-based social work has to offer should be well known both to in-patients and to health service colleagues.

A positive contribution at best

Connor and Tibbitt's study (1988) showed that where (a) social workers are hospital-based, (b) staffing levels permit their being linked to specific wards, and (c) they see patients early in their stay, maintain contact as appropriate and have community services to draw on, a series of important benefits ensues. These result from social workers being able to augment patients' social and material resources, and include:

- rapid recognition and resolution of worrying care problems resulting from emergency admissions, for example where there are relatives reliant on in-patients as carers;
- patients' wishes having a more prominent place in treatment plans, through social workers' advocacy;
- a better chance of the emotional impact of profound ill health and its

consequences for others close to the patient being recognised and responded to; and
• worries about financial resources and future care being eased through the initiation of arrangements for home care and accommodation, and applications for additional financial benefits.

The value of such intervention has been confirmed by the most comprehensive survey to date of user and carer feedback on the overall experience of hospital social work, from those who have received its services (SSI 1993). Drawing on a sample of fifty-nine users and twenty-six carers across three authorities this survey found hospital social workers (HSWs) were described as:

> 'helpful and caring' ... able to 'put things into perspective' ... extremely knowledgeable about benefits, housing, residential care, and appropriate domicilary services. They were also good listeners ... Two-thirds of users and carers stated things would have turned out differently ... [without] the HSW. One user expressed the sentiments of many: '[HSWs] do provide a wonderful service – being in hospital is stressful enough without having extra problems.'
>
> (SSI 1993: 23).

Unfortunately, a series of constraints and limitations seriously undermines the value of what hospital social workers can offer in-patients.

Constraints on access

Both as a consequence and a form of rationing of underfunded social work services, access to hospital-based social work is severely limited. Far from being extended as a key referral point, ward-attached social work is threatened by organisational retreat. To manage the speed-up of work required to complete complex community care assessments within shorter hospital stays, and with no extra staff, duty or intake systems have replaced a ward presence (McLeod 1995a; personal communication Committee BASWHRSIG 1998).

Moreover, accounts of hospital social work consistently report failure to apprise in-patients and their carers of the presence and role of hospital-based social workers (Bywaters 1991; Marks 1992; SSI 1992a, 1992b, 1993, 1995a and 1995b): 'More than two-thirds of all users and carers interviewed did not receive any information either written or verbal describing what they could expect from HSS

[Hospital Social Services], their priorities, or how to gain access' (SSI 1993: 10). Not surprisingly, rates of self-referral are uniformly very low – a serious problem, because reliance on referral by other hospital colleagues (SSI 1998b) fails to operationalise the requirements of large numbers of patients, notably older patients (Marks 1992; McLeod 1995b; Neill and Williams 1992; SSI 1998b).

Research carried out by one of the authors (Bywaters and McLeod 1996b, McLeod 1997) showed that hospital social workers wanted service users to be well informed, through direct contact with them, and also favoured their gaining readier access to services; but still held to the system of obtaining referrals from colleagues as a means of rationing demand (Bywaters and McLeod 1996b, McLeod 1997).

A restricted response

Not only is access being curtailed, but workers' repertoire of practice is also being restricted, in particular by the demands of meeting community care assessments to assist patient 'throughput' (see below, pp 108–9; Health Policy Network 1996; Henwood *et al.* 1997; SSI 1998b). Rachman's study (1995) revealed that hospital social workers were now only spending one-fifth of their working hours in face-to-face contact with service users and carers, compared with one-third in the late 1980s. An SSI review (1995b) found that hospital social workers had had to sacrifice counselling because of the volume of assessment work. Consequently the chances of offering sensitive, informed support to in-patients facing a daunting range of problems has been reduced. Hospital social workers themselves are keenly aware of what is happening:

> 'It just seems crazy to me if you have counselling skills, but can't offer them. I mean you establish a relationship so that you can understand what they are experiencing.'
>
> (Rachman 1995: 166)

> 'I think for dying patients there is a role for social workers ... I do some counselling, but managers think that the time I spend on it could be used more efficiently doing assessments.'
>
> (Davies and Connolly 1995b: 369)

A variety of further forms of preventive work is also having to be abandoned. These include reminiscence therapy, home visits and, while working on general wards, building up expertise in relation to specific conditions such as dementia (Davies and Connolly 1995b). One SSD known to the authors has instructed members of its hospital social work teams that counselling and benefits advice cannot be counted as part of their workload; another has restricted counselling following drug overdoses to one contact with each patient concerned (personal communication, two hospital social work teams 1998).

The limited nature of anti-oppressive practice

The value of hospital-based social work's contribution to patients' well-being is further compromised by the limited attention paid to issues of discrimination (McLeod 1995a). The SSI reports (1992a, 1992b and 1993) found that members of minority ethnic groups had a disproportionately low take-up of hospital social work services, but in a context of little evidence of ethnic monitoring, inconsistent attention to anti-racist practice and training, and a lack of interpreting services. Where benefits advice was undertaken, expertise in dealing with complex welfare rights issues was lacking and the provision of expert back-up unreliable. Social work teams also failed to press hospital authorities, who provide their accommodation, to ensure that this was accessible to disabled users. 'At none of the hospitals was there a high profile given to the need for access for people with disabilities to the office' (SSI 1992a: 13). In addition, the invisibility of homophobia as a live practice issue is reflected in the absence of even a single reference to it in the SSI reports themselves (1992a, 1992b and 1993).

Beyond holistic?

A further entrenched tendency within hospital social work practice limits its impact on unequal social relations. With very few recorded exceptions, practice is both conceptualised and carried out on a one-to-one basis. The tradition of taking a 'holistic' approach, of trying to address the 'psychosocial implications of the impact of the illness, disability or loss'(Badawi and Biamonti 1990: 38), continues today (Rachman 1995). But it is almost exclusively confined to the definition of (and response to) physical, psychological, social and material issues as constituting *an individual's own problems* or, at most, problems that involve only their immediate family.

Hospital social workers are not geared to identifying, researching and servicing the collective interests of hospital patients as populations or interest groups. Consequently the weight of their organising potential has not been thrown behind the identification and raising of issues of critical importance to patients' well-being, such as the shortages reflected in the inadequate feeding, general care and high rates of infection discussed earlier in this chapter (pp 98–9). As one of the authors has argued, 'Working for change in the hospital setting may require more of the skills of a community worker than a caseworker' (Bywaters 1986: 672). The benefits of a more collective approach are epitomised in the following examples:

- Concerned at the unstimulating environment faced by older patients on a rehabilitation ward, the lack of feedback to staff on quality of care and the inhibitions faced by individual patients in providing this, Clarke (1993), a primary nurse on the ward, set up, with the patients' agreement, a discussion and feedback group. The upshot was that 'patients sparked each other off' (1993: 44) and several significant issues concerning day-to-day care were raised and then put to the relevant staff. These included changes to improve the meal service (taken up by catering staff and nurses); improvements to the heating system on the ward; and the dangerous inaccessibility of pull-cords (both issues subsequently addressed by the operations and maintenance manager).
- When hospital social worker members of BASWHRSIG from around the country reported concerns that numbers of gravely ill patients with only a few days to live were being shunted out of hospital into nursing homes, the committee of BASWHRSIG raised the issue with the BMA (McLeod 1995a). This contributed to a rising tide of public disquiet, leading to the Department of Health issuing guidance on the issue (NHS Executive 1995).
- To establish the extent to which patients were informed about hospital-based social work services, as a preliminary to a project addressing questions of access, the patient population of two elderly services wards were asked at two-monthly intervals whether they knew that there were hospital social workers on site and what services these might offer. The results of this 'community profiling' approach (Green 1997) were a revelation to the social work team members, as around three-quarters of the patients (73 per cent) did not even know there were hospital social workers present (McLeod 1995b).

From hierarchy to co-operative?

Working relations with other hospital colleagues constitute the remaining problematic dimension to hospital-based social work's contribution to in-patient well-being. Hospital-based social work presents only a muted challenge to the hierarchical medical behaviour which, as we saw earlier in this chapter, runs counter to in-patients' interests (pp 99–100). Although at times hospital social workers do manage to act as advocates, representing patients' interests in treatment options (Connor and Tibbitt 1988) and negotiating some extensions of in-patient stays in order to set up more adequate post-discharge arrangements, and although hospital doctors now identify social work input as intrinsic to achieving a decent level of patient care by a multidisciplinary team (Davies and Connolly 1995a), nevertheless doctors still commonly assume that social work input should be on *their* terms (Davies and Connolly 1995a).

This situation does not reflect hospital social workers' lack of professional nerve, but the unequal nature of the power relations involved. As Kendrick (1995a) has argued, working relations between doctors and non-medical colleagues are imbued with the power differences of class and status (Williams and Calnan 1996; Gabe *et al.* 1994; Stacey 1988). These foster and legitimise doctors' propensity to command, reinforced by a lack of assertiveness on the part of less privileged occupational groups (Kendrick 1995b). Despite the pressures of inadequate funding and rising managerialism (Health Policy Network 1995), doctors' social advantage continues to be institutionalised *vis-à-vis* other health care colleagues in the hospital system. As Mackay *et al.* (1995: 8) argue: 'It is doctors who retain final and legal responsibility for patients. Doctors enjoy undoubted supremacy in the management and direction of the health care team. Without doctors' goodwill to listen, the contributions of other professionals can be marginalised.'

These subordinating influences are compounded by the gendered nature of doctor–social worker relations. In contrast to consultants, hospital social workers are predominantly women (SSI 1992a), clustered in the lower reaches of a profession with relatively low pay and professional status (Mullender and Perrott 1998). Not surprisingly, observations of ward meetings across a range of specialisms found evidence in discussions between consultants and social workers of a 'subordinating dynamic based on gender' (Penhale 1997: 50).

Such entrenched structural problems require profound solutions. In the shorter term, first, a growing number of hospital doctors – albeit most frequently in specialties such as geriatrics and paediatrics – who also link health problems with social disadvantage, have embarked on power-sharing initiatives not just with hospital social work colleagues but also with patients and carers; see, for example, O'Neill 1996 and Spencer 1996. O'Neill has instituted training for non-social work colleagues in the geriatric health care team about the appropriate grounds for referral to hospital social workers, and run informal training programmes for carers in order to disseminate information about recovery from stroke and the development of dementia. Second, in the wake of public outcry and professional concern about the failure of the medical profession to monitor itself effectively in relation to differential risks of cardiac surgery performed by different surgeons (Treasure 1998), a more systematic, ongoing, independent system for reviewing doctors' performance is being brought in through professional and governmental action (Smith 1998; NHS Executive 1998). Within the medical profession itself this move towards higher public accountability has been recognised as a critical juncture in giving doctor–patient power relations a more democratic tilt (Smith 1998).

There is evidence of hospital social workers allying themselves with nursing staff to circumvent consultants' powers, in the interests of meeting patients' social care needs (Henwood *et al.* 1997). However, working relations between social work and nursing staff are threatened to the extent that the two professions now compete for the same 'territory', with nurses moving into counselling (Burnard 1995; Jones 1997; Wesson 1997), care management (Naylor 1990; Schurdell *et al.* 1995) and community liaison (Mayor 1995). As yet the coverage provided by nurses who occupy such roles is patchy (Naish 1995), and limited by staff shortages, cutbacks in nursing (Mark 1996) and the institutional role given to SSDs in assessment and care management. Nevertheless, the drive in nursing for enhanced professional status through assuming social work roles is liable to institutionalise conflict between social workers and nurses (Bywaters 1989).

DISCHARGE PLANNING: CONVALESCENCE AND
CONTINUING CARE

Introduction

Hospital-based social workers' contribution to in-patients' well-being may be heavily circumscribed, but their role in discharge planning remains centre stage. As the SSI puts it, 'SSDs need to recognise ... hospital social workers as key players in the arranging and purchasing of care' (1995b: 2). In this section we identify the main policy developments currently informing discharge planning and the service provision it feeds into. We then examine the major consequences for hospital patients and hospital-based social workers caught up in undemocratic discharge planning procedures, insufficient facilities for convalescence and recovery, questionable aspects of transfer to residential care and the inequities of means-testing.

Shifting the responsibility for care

Critical events still shaping discharge planning, convalescence and continuing care occurred across the life of the previous political administration. Most crucial was the dramatic decrease in the number of acute, convalescent and continuing care beds, accompanied by increased 'productivity'. Between 1982 and 1993 there was a 23 per cent reduction in general and acute hospital beds, a 65 per cent increase in 'throughput' and a 160 per cent increase in day cases. These trends were even more pronounced in geriatric care, with a 29 per cent reduction in general and acute beds, an 149 per cent increase in throughput and a 700 per cent increase in day cases (Henwood 1995). This was accompanied by a 38 per cent reduction in continuing care beds for older people between 1983 and 1996 (Audit Commission 1997) and a 45 per cent reduction in the average length of stay in geriatric specialties, from thirty-six days in 1989/90 to twenty days in 1994/5 (Audit Commission 1997).

Admittedly, these events coincided with the development and adoption of various new technologies and treatment regimes. Day surgery, minimal access ('keyhole') surgery and 'hospital at home' (the relocation of medical/nursing procedures to home settings) were all enthusiastically endorsed by the medical profession, patients and the manufacturers of the technology involved (Henwood 1995). But the mainspring of the speed-up of hospital care was cost-cutting, linked to an ideological commitment to the creation of an internal market in health care, the development of the independent sector in social care provision, and the promotion of individual 'self-sufficiency' (Means and Smith 1994; Mohan 1995).

The withdrawal of the NHS from the provision of continuing care free at the point of use was subsequently subject to legal challenge (Audit Commission 1997), but the die had been cast. Not only had the NHS retreated from provision for convalescence and rehabilitation (Marks 1992) but, as the House of Commons Select Committee on Health (1996) commented, a situation had been created 'in which general, as distinct from specialist long-term nursing care is no longer considered to be an NHS responsibility, but rather as social care and thus eligible for means testing' (quoted in Audit Commission 1997: 12).

A new deal?

Under the current government the abolition of the internal market in the NHS is seen amongst other things as relieving the pressure on hospitals to cultivate high rates of throughput of patients as the benchmark of efficiency (DoH 1997a); and, as previously discussed, pressure on NHS hospital resources has been relieved to some degree by additional government funding (see Chapter 2). The forthcoming white paper on continuing care has been trailed as removing charges for the health care element of care, in non-hospital settings (*Independent on Sunday*, 17 January 1999: 1). Nevertheless, the current government's approach to recovery or long-term care seems revisionist, rather than being characterised by a shift back to the principles of universal state-funded short- or long-term provision free at the point of use. The major focus is on making better use of existing resources, through improved co-ordination and planning between NHS and social services (DoH 1997a), and on exploring more 'cost-effective' alternatives to residential, nursing home or acute hospital bed use, including schemes to divert hospital patients from admission (Audit Commission 1997) or from residential or nursing home care after discharge (DoH 1997a). The assumptions of the review into long-term care are encapsulated in the following:

> Such a review might address the issue of how far the state has a responsibility to support individuals, and how far individuals should plan for their own needs. At present each generation pays for the

previous one through taxation. This may no longer be sustainable as the population of economically active people shrinks over the next 40–50 years and the number of people over 75 and 85 grows.

(Audit Commission 1997: 83)

We now turn to the major consequences of this policy context for the equitable chances of returning health or continuing well-being of those patients being discharged from hospital, and social work's role in these.

Stacking the odds against recovery and continuing health

Problematic involvement in assessment for care on discharge

The constraints on in-patients' access to hospital social work services are reflected in evidence of low levels of assessment for care on discharge. Two years after the implementation of the NHS and Community Care Act, 40 per cent of older patients in a Community Health Councils' study said that no member of staff had discussed with them the sort of help they might need after leaving hospital (Association of Community Health Councils for England and Wales (ACHCEW) 1996). Furthermore, one of the authors (McLeod 1995b) uncovered evidence in an acute elderly services hospital unit that crucial requirements for care, with consequences for health in the long term, were being missed. Even when hospital patients' post-discharge needs *are* considered, hierarchical and discriminatory practices often deny them the opportunity to shape decisions in their own interests. Hospital patients are not routinely involved in multidisciplinary care planning meetings (Godfrey and Moore 1996; McLeod 1995a; SSI 1993 and 1998b), and the SSI found that fewer than 25 per cent of patients were even aware these meetings were being held (1993). Moreover, analysis of ward-level inter-professional discharge planning meetings suggests a continuing tendency for hospital social workers and health colleagues to compete in passing the buck in the face of resources shortages (Chadwick and Russell 1989; Neill and Williams 1992; McLeod 1995b). There is no guarantee that patients will receive written copies of care plans (Audit Commission 1997; SSI 1993 and 1998b). In Godfrey and Moore's study (1996) a variety of hospital medical and social work staff in different specialisms genuinely thought they did involve users and carers in assessment; yet 'there [was] ... in all accounts, from older people in particular, a pervasive sense of powerlessness within the hospital, a fear that "they" will decide the person cannot go home' (1996: 38). And despite carers' entitlement under the Carers (Recognition and Services) Act 1995, carers' assessments rarely occur (SSI 1998b).

Measures to ensure that patients from minority ethnic groups or with a range of impairments can participate fully in assessment also remain haphazard. There is an official commitment to using interpreting services, but staff have still been relying to a considerable extent on family members and hospital staff not designated or trained for this work (SSI 1993). Notwithstanding a consistent pattern of high rates of sensory, cognitive or multiple impairment across older patient populations, basic communication aids such as 'communicators' to amplify speech, leaflets in large print, information on audiotape or contact with advocacy services are not routinely available (McLeod 1997).

Getting better at home? Insufficient facilities for convalescence and recovery

Following discharge from hospital, the NHS retreat from provision for convalescence or recovery, coupled with inadequate substitute social services resources, has worrying consequences for health. Paradoxically it has led to a proportion of patients continuing to receive expensive and inappropriate acute in-patient care, instead of convalescence or remedial treatment. The Audit Commission (1997) suggests that this could account for nearly 20 per cent of unnecessary lengths of stay in acute hospitals. Henwood *et al.*'s study of interagency collaboration in discharge planning across six localities also found that, in half, 'budgetary constraints were creating serious impediments to the speed at which social services were able to facilitate patient discharge' (1997: 44).

In increasing numbers patients are being discharged precipitately without sufficient support. Henwood *et al.* found evidence of routine discharge of patients 'who may not be acutely ill, but are not actually well' (1997: 37), with hospital staff concerned about their well-being. Particularly vulnerable are older people who frequently live alone, are likely to be grappling with a range of health problems and impairment and, due to poverty, cannot readily fund the material conditions to underwrite recovery at home, such as adequate heating or a tele-phone (Arber and Ginn 1995).

Henwood's earlier study (1995) showed that even when treatments such as day surgery, minimal access surgery (MAS) and 'hospital at home' are specifically designed to relocate recovery at home, in the absence of appropriate support from public services they make heavy demands on both ex-patients and relatives. These include worrying gaps in the provision of pain relief; inappropriate emotional and phys-ical demands arising from what amounts to maintaining an intensive care environment with round-the-clock nursing; and the stresses of longer-term care, involving dealing with bedsores and bathing.

When short-term packages of care are provided through discharge planning, there are widespread reports of key provisions being in short supply: night sitting, home care, short periods of intensive home care, help with transport, shopping, laundry, residential convalescent facilities and companionship (Age Concern London, 1995; Clark *et al.* 1996; Harding 1997; McLeod 1995a; personal communication BASWHRSIG committee 1998; SSI 1998b; Waddington and Henwood 1996). Moreover, there are accounts of hospital social workers maintaining covert contact with ex-patients beyond organi-sationally sanctioned time-limits, to ensure that appropriate services actually are going in and to offer further psychological support (personal communication BASWHRSIG committee 1998).

Evidence from descriptive and controlled studies demonstrates that when sufficiently comprehensive and timely residential and home care facilities are supplied to aid recovery and convalescence, then dramatic health-promoting benefits occur. A study of Outlands, an SSD rehabilitation unit in Devon, considered outcomes after a maxi-mum six-week stay and found:

> despite the fact that all residents were considered in need of residen-tial care on admission ... three-quarters returned to their own homes at the end of their rehabilitation episode. Moreover half of these needed no ongoing social services support on discharge at all.
>
> (Wistow and Lewis 1996: 38)

Waddington and Henwood's (1996) account of eighteen British Red Cross 'Home from Hospital' schemes around the country drew on ex-patients' evaluations. The scheme offers volunteer support averag-ing six home visits for up to four weeks following discharge and pro-vides help with the activities of daily living for (mostly older) people living alone. Beneficiaries' reports indicated that it had helped with cleaning, cooking and shopping to a far more substantial degree than had statutory services, and also that 'only 6 per cent believed they received companionship from statutory services' (1996: 67) as compared with 73 per cent from the Home from Hospital scheme. The critical difference for health and well-being which such practical and personal support offers shines out: '"It helps you get better when you don't have to struggle to do everything ..."; "It was wonderful. I was scared of coming home by myself, but each morning I awoke and remembered that [the volunteer] would be along soon"' (Waddington and Henwood 1996: 93).

Controlled studies by Townsend *et al.* (1988 and 1992) confirm this picture, revealing long-term health benefits. Older patients in the experimental group received home care support for up to twelve hours a week for two weeks following discharge in addition to the standard statutory provision available to both groups. The home care involved (a) practical care; (b) encouraging and helping towards independence and (c) organising the necessary support from statutory services, or else help from family and friends and neighbours (Townsend *et al.* 1992: 137). Across the following eighteen months members of the experimental group were significantly less likely to be readmitted as an emergency admission, experience multiple readmissions or to spend as much time in hospital following readmission (Townsend *et al.* 1992). Differences in readmission rates were most marked amongst patients living alone and aged over 85.

These initiatives point to the benefits for patients, carers, the NHS and social services which could accrue if funding were to be released so that comprehensive services are available on discharge. As Henwood and colleagues argue, 'ways must be found to ensure local initiatives and good practice become routine and are absorbed into the mainstream throughout the country' (1997: 7). Moreover, although short-term input may hold long-term health benefits, the goal of equal chances of health maintenance requires the continuance of substantial levels of care beyond short-term schemes. This was a concern of many Red Cross volunteers: '"There are many people living alone with no close family nearby desperately in need of help of a very basic kind. One wonders what happens to these people when their volunteer finishes ..."' (Waddington and Henwood 1996: 43).

Finally, the shortfall in social services and health service input is implicated in unplanned, emergency readmissions on a vast scale: 23,340 patients aged over 75 were readmitted as an emergency within twenty-eight days of discharge between July and September 1996 (Hansard 1997). Given the impact of winter on admissions, a staggering figure of about 100,000 patients a year over 75 being readmitted within a month as emergencies is a realistic extrapolation (Harding 1997). It is reasonable to conclude that pressure to save resources by discharging early from hospital, combined with insufficient care in the community, contributes to this harrowing situation.

Safe at last? Discharge to residential or nursing home care

Tilting the odds

The shortcomings of discharge planning also form part of a complex matrix of factors which raise the odds of inappropriate entry to residential or nursing home care. In its follow-up inspection of the discharge of older people from hospital to residential or nursing home care, the SSI (1995b) found that 'living alone' and 'falling' were considered the major risk factors influencing a recommendation of residential care by hospital-based social workers. As Harding (1997) has shown, underprovision of safe, very sheltered housing with home care back-up where necessary and cutbacks in primary care services such as chiropody have a major part to play in creating both of these health hazards.

Perverse funding incentives are also continuing to drive movement from hospital into residential care on financial grounds. Taking residential allowances and income from the sale of people's homes into account can mean that the net cost of residential as opposed to domiciliary care is cheaper to local authorities (Audit Commission 1997). Moreover, the supply of nursing home places in an area is significantly related to higher rates of discharge from hospital to those homes, while the volume of money tied up in residential care in a situation of financial stringency restricts funds for developing intensive home care alternatives (Audit Commission 1997).

The current pressure on hospital social workers to carry out complex care assessments at speed and withdraw from counselling may also lead to inappropriate residential placements. Wistow and Lewis (1996: 37–8) have highlighted the significance of the Department of Health's finding that the crucial factor influencing people's decision to stay at home with a package of community care services was not 'dependency level' but motivation, with 'fear of loneliness, of being a burden' making entry to care more likely. 'Sheer determination' to stay put was the most striking feature of people who chose to stay at home. As Wistow and Lewis argue, 'such research would suggest that care plans or interventions which are geared towards tackling these psychological issues may be more effective at reducing admissions to institutional care than those which focus solely on mental or physical symptoms'.

Participation in planning for residential care

Even if residential or nursing home care is appropriate, the chances that patients will actively choose the home are slim. While carers and relatives for the most part took the initiative in checking out residential accommodation, the SSI (1995b) found across two inspections that only limited information – sometimes no more than a list – was made available by SSDs to assist users and carers in making their choice. Users rarely visited. Although infirmity or ill health were given as the reason, the Inspectorate found no instances of weekend or overnight trial stays being available. In most cases a maximum of two homes was considered, in 26 per cent of cases only one, shedding a different light on the finding that 80 per cent of patients reported having their first choice. Attention to the specific requirements of members of minority ethnic groups was also not in evidence.

Once admitted to residential care, documentation on patients' individual health and care requirements can be haphazard – reflecting badly not only on social work input, but on that of the multidiscipinary team as a whole. Bennet et al.'s (1995) survey of older people in nursing homes after assessment found 'no social information for 20 per cent, no nursing information for 35 per cent and no physiotherapy information for 90 per cent' (quoted in Audit Commission 1997: 23). This pattern was confirmed in Henwood et al.'s multi-locality study (1997) and in an SSI inspection (1998b). Such shortcomings are all the more worrying in a situation in which systematic and comprehensive medical care of older people in residential and nursing homes has yet to be organised (Black and Bowman 1997).

Taken together, these circumstances point to the importance of the post-admission review as a fail-safe mechanism to protect older peoples' interests. But the SSI (1995a and 1995b) found that it could not be relied upon. Instead, the residential placement rapidly became a *fait accompli.* Although reviews were usually occurring after four to six weeks, they were largely about confirming the placement. There was little evidence of a reassessment of progress or emphasis on rehabilitation. Care managers were rarely significantly involved beyond the six-weekly review. Other than in one local authority, there was seldom any subsequent review.

'The final turn of the screw'

The administration of means-testing for continuing care, previously free when provided by the NHS, remains integral to hospital social workers' involvement in discharge planning. The inequity of this situation has already been highlighted and continues to be the subject of legal challenge (House of Commons Health Committee 1996; *Independent on Sunday* 9 November 1997: 2). Two serious health consequences can ensue. First, it can rapidly have dire effects on the fundamentals of physical and emotional well-being of those on a moderate income. These are illustrated in a test case in Buckinghamshire to oppose moves by the local authority to evict the son of a woman whose savings had been exhausted in paying for nursing home care, so that the family home could be sold to meet continuing fees (*Independent on Sunday* 9 November 1997: 2). Second, in the longer term, as Challis and Henwood have argued, stripping down older people's assets may lessen their chances of informal family care: 'It would be naive to assume that the removal of the prospect of inheritance will have no effect on future generations' willingness to bear the expense and take on the responsibility of caring for dependent relatives' (1994: 1498).

The preceding discussion of in-patient experience, discharge and aftercare has shown that social work is both up against and implicated in many barriers to a more equal chance of health. But our analysis also points to a series of measures that would develop social work's contribution and we conclude by discussing these. In doing so we do not disaggregate the different stages of the hospitalisation process, as more effective practice at one stage holds benefits for practice throughout.

MAKING IT BETTER: SOCIAL WORK, HOSPITALISATION, AND A MORE EQUAL CHANCE OF HEALTH

Redistributing socio-economic resources

The starting point of most discussions about how hospital social work might feed into a more equitable experience of health is the reorganisation of the NHS–SSD boundary (see Audit Commission 1997; Henwood 1997). But we begin by taking a step back from this.

At its inception, it was hoped that by offering fairer access to health care the NHS would contribute to gradually reducing the incidence of ill health in the population, so that in time there would be proportionately fewer claims on its services (Jones 1994). We now know that this was not to be (Davey Smith *et al.* 1990). The primary means of reducing overload on hospital care and giving it the best chance of contributing to a fair chance of health is not through NHS (or SSD) provision but through equalising people's access to socio-economic resources in the community. In our analysis, for example, it was the socially disadvantaged position of relatively poor older people which was implicated in their disproportionate re-entry into NHS hospital care for treatment, greater vulnerability to treatments' shortcomings, and risk of being short-changed over convalescence or continuing care. Behind this scenario lay a range of socio-economic conditions known to be associated with increased chances of ill health, including low incomes, poor housing and social isolation (Wistow and Lewis 1996), together with discriminatory assumptions about the acceptability of ill health and imminent death (O'Neill 1996).Though more equitable chances of health can accrue from changes to organisational funding and policy and to social work practice in hospital, these will be hidebound to the extent that central and local government fail to take redistributive action on access to social and material resources in daily life.

Better-funded services, free at the point of use

Meanwhile, both NHS and social services provision do require substantially higher levels of funding in their own right; but also if provision is to be accessible on an equitable basis, to be free at the point of use. Public debate on these issues centres on the overwhelming and politically unacceptable scale of the income tax increases that would be required, together with the spectre of the uncontrollable demands of servicing the needs of an ageing population (Harding *et al.* 1996). The alarmist and repressive nature of both standpoints is revealed through the following two alternative positions that have been put forward.

- The BMA's review of options to meet NHS funding requirements more adequately, that is, to put the NHS on a par with the per capita spending of OECD comparators (see Chapter 2), shows that obtaining such funding through general taxation is a pragmatic possibility. The amounts required per annum are *less* than the previous government's income tax *cuts* for a full year in its final budget (BMA 1997).
- Harding *et al.*'s (1996) analysis acknowledges that long-term care costs will rise as the population ages, but shows that until 2030 these are unlikely to constitute a greater proportion of public expenditure than across the 1980s to late 1990s, a period of public expenditure constraint. On these grounds too, higher investment through general taxation to ensure a more decent level of care and greater equity in its accessibility should not be assumed to equate with public expenditure ballooning out of control.

Two profound constraints on measures for more equitable health care remain untouched by this discussion: the inflationary pressures on NHS funding of the pharmaceutical and medical technology industries, and the continued presence of private health care (see Chapter 2). The fundamental inequity of the two-tier private/public system for NHS hospital patients has been apparent in this chapter. However, ending private health care is not central to the government's agenda (DoH 1997a). Moreover, it is grappling with a large-scale problem of dilapidated hospital buildings, exacerbated by financial neglect under the previous administration (Butler 1998). An NHS estates estimate suggests that 'the repairs bill is equal to some 15 per cent of the total value of NHS buildings, said to be £20 billion' (Butler 1998:23). Faced with this task and anxious to maintain fiscal 'prudence', the government has relied heavily on the Private Finance Initiative (PFI) to fund investment in hospital plant, thereby avoiding outlays classed as public expenditure (BMA 1997). However, the longer-term risks include not only higher overall costs for the exchequer due to the higher borrowing costs incurred by the private sector being passed on through leasehold arrangements, but also the growth of privatisation in health care, as ownership of the hospitals remains within the private sector (Whitfield 1997).

Organisational developments

Complementing these developments, a series of changes in the NHS and social services organisational backdrop to hospital social work are essential to more equitable chances of health.

Performance measurement: Shifting from throughput to quality of care as the benchmark

The government's stated aims are to move from a market-oriented measurement of hospital performance to one more concerned with quality of care, discernible to patients and GP referrers alike: 'Under the NHS internal market, performance was driven by what could readily be measured: the financial bottom line and the numbers of "finished consultant episodes"' (DoH 1997a: 63). This should pave the way for treatment regimes which fit patients' health requirements rather than vice versa (1997a: 64):

> Fair access must be to care that is effective, appropriate and timely, and complies with agreed standards. For example, increasing provision of treatments proven to bring benefit such as hip replacements, *provision of rehabilitation at the point when it can offer most benefit, sustained delivery of health and social care to those with long-term needs* [our emphasis] and reducing inappropriate treatments.

The chances of the government putting such plans into action are inextricable from funding increases. Nevertheless, the development of Primary Care Groups and organisations representing patients' interests (discussed below) may sustain pressure to bring the government's practice closer to its own vision. What this change of standpoint offers is a chance of refocusing concern on the quality of patients' long-term health careers, as opposed to speeding them through the hospital system. It would mean, for example, reopening closed wards as convalescent facilities; nursing home accommodation being taken over by the NHS as model convalescent centres free at the point of need; greater use of respite care to meet patients' as well as carers' needs. It would also mean developing facilities for more extensive provision of intensive home care, not only to reduce admissions but to provide a decent chance of recovery afterwards. It is only as such a range of resources becomes available that hospital social workers will be rescued from the health-damaging job (Rachman 1995) of means-testing and rationing inadequate resources.

Mapping demand and service provision

Nothing we have argued so far obviates the need for informed and economical deployment of services. As the Audit Commission (1997) has proposed, both local health authorities and SSDs need to undertake more comprehensive mapping of the supply of and demand for services. It is, perhaps, an example of institutionalised ageism that the Audit Commission found that social services did not record 'the proportion of placements to nursing homes or residential homes from each local hospital' (1997: 55) and that although all health authorities had policies and criteria for continuing care, only about 45 per cent had mapped continuing care needs or the current number of beds available. Henwood *et al.*'s survey (1997) of Health Authority–social services collaboration and the SSI follow-up survey of discharge planning (1998b) both showed that, for the most part, joint or integrated commissioning strategies for continuing health and social care were still lacking.

Developing a hospital-based social work presence

Our analysis also reveals the strategic importance of hospital-based social workers for access to and the deployment of social services provision. More generous staffing levels, underwritten by a higher management profile within SSDs, would support the development of ward- and clinic-based attachments to facilitate more equitable and timely access, improvements in in-patient care, more comprehensive and uniformly available discharge planning and longer-term post-discharge care – all relieving patients from unnecessary suffering.

Developing the means of representing hospital patients' interests

Throughout our account, however, it has been clear that hospital patients are repeatedly not treated as co-workers by NHS staff or by social workers. Hospital-based social workers therefore cannot simplistically be relied upon to champion patients' social care requirements over against vested departmental and professional interests. Means of representing and asserting patients' interests have to be sought, to counterbalance defensive practice. The NHS publication 'A First-class Service' incorporates user/patient representation in the National Institute for Clinical Excellence (NICE) and a National Survey of Patient and User Experience, as a means of gaining patients' views in the development of hospital care (NHS Executive 1998). But our analysis suggests that a more active and ground-level, as well as independent and combative, approach is required.

Coote and Hunter (1996) have identified four promising strategies along these lines:

- more explicit recognition of NHS patients' substantive and procedural rights, backed by tighter legal enforcement;
- a greater role for local authorities in commissioning health services, as being to some extent democratic bodies representing the interests of patients as citizens;
- self-help interest groups initiatives, such as those representing women's interests in childbirth, that exert some leverage on services' responsiveness (Doyal 1995); and
- the development of the powers of Community Health Councils (CHCs).

As Coote and Hunter admit, current CHC capacity for influential and independent representation is circumscribed by limited powers to hold health authorities to account, by limited administrative resources and by the predominance of a white, middle-class membership. Nevertheless, in a revised and developed form CHCs could offer a good representative organisational model. As Coote and Hunter argue (1996: 88):

> Suitably reformed and resourced CHCs could perform a useful role as lay experts representing local interests in the commissioning of health services. This would entail increased funding, membership selection independent of the NHS and rights to information, to be consulted, to inspect, to counsel and represent individuals.

Our account has already reflected CHCs' potential in relation to the issue of malnutrition in hospital. It was the ACHCEW report 'Hungry in Hospital' (1997) which raised the question of inadequate feeding of hospital patients as a public issue, and resulted in the United Kingdom Central Council – nursing's regulatory body – writing to all hospitals to make it clear that nurses have professional obligations to meet patients' nutritional needs (*Guardian* Society 14 May 1997: 7), thereby adding greater pressure for action on the issue.

Logistical problems concerning the representation of hospital inpatients' and ex-patients' interests remain. The point of greatest vulnerability may coincide with such profound ill health or social crisis that individual challenge or protest is not feasible; the requirements and social situations of patients are very diverse, and the episodic nature of hospital treatment and the geographical scatter of patients' homes make it difficult to assemble the views of a representative cross-section. The following voluntary sector initiatives provide possible solutions to these difficulties. First, the Alzheimer's Disease Society has been able to develop advocacy networks, with a brief to represent patients' interests on wards, independently of health and social work professionals (Killeen 1996). Second, deficiencies in care and resource provision for disadvantaged groups have been publicised. For example, Help the Aged, as an organisation representing the interests of older people, brought the shocking figures concerning rates of emergency readmissions for older patients into the spotlight of the press (Harding 1997). Help the Aged was also a leading player in the campaign to address inadequate standards of care of older people in NHS hospitals. This resulted in the government instituting an inquiry into this issue (HAS 2000 1998), to be followed by a national service framework setting hospital care standards for older people (Warden 1998). Third, focus group research, independent of the NHS, drawing on feedback from patients' experience of the whole hospitalisation process, has enabled views from geographically and socially diverse groups of patients to be gathered, synthesised and published in a form which has both the legitimacy and protection of representative collective feedback (Tritter 1996).

Re-forming professional practice

To the extent that the major developments in resource distribution, policy, organisational frameworks and activism which we have outlined come into being, social work concerned with hospitalisation will be freed to fulfil its potential to enhance not subvert health. But two further internal transformations in day-to-day practice have emerged as necessary to combating health inequalities. First, hospital-based social workers need to engage more directly and broadly in tackling discrimination amongst the patient population. Second, if issues of fundamental importance to health are not to be missed, practice needs to be based on analysing and responding to problems on a collective and strategic basis.

As regards the evolution of hospital multidisciplinary practice into co-operative, egalitarian health care incorporating social workers and patients as co-workers on an equal footing, our conclusions remain at worst pessimistic; at best, cautious. The development of more democratic working relations on the part of doctors is under way and carrying governmental endorsement, but is still limited. The potential for alliances between social workers and nurses remains threatened by sectional interests. Co-working with patients, as health workers in their own right, and explicitly tackling the inequalities in health that beset them, arguably provides the best basis for collaborative working.

Hospital social work is of strategic importance to well-being, but currently beleaguered by a set of powerful constraints. Underpinned by major policy changes, adequately resourced, held to account by more robust, independent representation of patients' interests and refocused on more truly co-operative anti-oppressive and collective strategies, it has the chance to fulfil its potential.

Chapter 6

Facing death

INTRODUCTION

The advent of the hospice movement and the growth of palliative care have played a major part in changing the disablist situation where having a life-threatening illness[5] and becoming terminally ill were accepted as necessarily accompanied by a decline in the quality of life. The evolution of palliative care has made more effective pain relief available (Working Party on Clinical Guidelines in Palliative Care (WPCGPC) 1998) and stimulated the development of better relief of other distressing symptoms such as unremitting nausea, vomiting and muscle spasms (Williams and Corcoran 1996). The influence of the 'hospice model' has also produced improved responses to the psychosocial requirements of people living with life-threatening illness. For example, the generalised conspiracy of silence in the health care system which condemned people who were dying to be unapprised of the fact of their own imminent death – leaving them powerless to take informed decisions about the remainder of their life – has largely been breached (Seale 1989; Sheldon 1997). Recognition that people with life-threatening illness and those close to them may be grappling with 'total pain' ('a complex of physical, emotional, social and spiritual elements', Saunders 1996: 1600) has informed the development of palliative care, moving it beyond a narrow 'medical model'.

This is reflected in the World Health Organisation's (1990) definition of palliative care:

> Palliative care is the active total care of patients and their families by a multiprofessional team when the patient's disease is no longer

responsive to curative treatment. Control of pain, of other symptoms and of psychological, social and spiritual problems is paramount. The goal of palliative care[6] is the achievement of good quality of life for patients and their families. Many aspects of palliative care are also applicable earlier in the course of illness.

(cited in Oliviere *et al.* 1998: 2)

One consequence of this development is that in hospice care, professional social workers' input has been legitimised as more central to the professional team than is the case in other health care settings (Oliviere *et al.* 1998). Indeed Cicely Saunders, who has been an outstanding activist and driving force in the development of palliative care, should be reclaimed as a pioneering social work figure. In her early career she trained not only as a nurse and subsequently a doctor, but as a social worker – becoming a 'lady almoner' at St Thomas's Hospital. It was from listening to individual users' accounts that she identified general social problems which needed to be addressed: '"It was in my social worker days that I continually met patients who showed me how much needed to be done in the control of pain and the understanding of dying patients and their families"' (quoted in Kastenbaum 1993: 263).

Today palliative care has a substantial presence in British health care, with 228 in-patient units, approximately 500 community-based palliative care teams, 250 day centres and about 350 hospitals with palliative care support teams or nurses (Jackson and Eve 1998). It has become a medical specialism (Ahmedzai and Biswas 1993). Its approach has been espoused by the World Health Organisation and, in a variety of organisational forms, it is now a global phenomenon (Hockley 1997).

Despite these major developments, this chapter will show that even when death threatens, the experience of illness in Britain reflects and perpetuates social inequalities. Medical and pharmacological relief of symptoms still has far to go (see, for example, WPCGPC 1998). The state of evidence on the benefits or drawbacks of existing forms of palliative care remains problematic. However, as we outline, the provision of material and social resources, of treatment and social work for people with life-threatening illness that is potentially available is far from comprehensive, and is marked by social divisions within the population concerned. As with the other aspects of the experience of illness discussed in Chapters 4 and 5, this represents a situation of socially constructed disadvantage and unnecessary, inequitable suffering.

Several aspects of current government policy reflect awareness of such inequalities in the experience of dying. However, we show that the unequal distribution of material and social resources refracted through government policy as a whole, as well as through policy directly concerning health care, social care and palliative care, is implicated in widespread suffering amongst people with life-threatening illness. Their position is also marginalised in professional social work generally. We argue that these inequalities constitute a human rights issue, requiring as they do a focus on redressing existing dimensions to inequality. We conclude by examining one of the most promising recent developments for bringing this about: a series of diverse initiatives characteried by collective lay activism, involving some professional support. In an incremental way, these have begun to refashion the power relations shaping life-threatening illness in the interests of the people concerned and disadvantaged groups within this population. As such they share the hallmarks of progressive social work for health identified in earlier chapters.[7]

THE BENEFITS OF PALLIATIVE CARE: PROBLEMS OF EVIDENCE

Indicative, not conclusive

Evidence for whether or not intervention by specialist palliative care teams produces more positive outcomes than conventional health and social care services has been reviewed by Hearn and Higginson (1998). Drawing on research world-wide and focusing on services 'leading the field', the teams they studied were typically composed of 'doctors, clinical nurse specialists, social workers, chaplains, therapists and psychologists or psychiatrists' (1998: 317, 318). Whether community-, hospital- or hospice-based, each team's key aims (1998: 319) were to:

- plan and implement effective integrated treatment and care;
- communicate effectively with the patient, with all other professionals and agencies involved in the care of the patient and within itself; and
- audit its activities and outcomes.

The work of such teams was characterised by improved outcomes in important respects: symptom control, patient and carer satisfaction with care, patients being able to spend more time at home and being more likely to die in their preferred location. Nevertheless, Hearn and Higginson strike some cautionary notes on the validity of the evidence. Only a minority of studies took the form of randomised controlled trials, and separating the positive effects of constituent members' work from the approach of the team as a whole is difficult.

Dearth of systematic evidence on social work

The absence of systematic evidence on the benefits of social work input into hospice-based palliative care teams, the site of social work's most explicit and concentrated engagement in palliative care, is even more marked. This may reflect its lower status in the professional hierarchies involved. Even major recent edited texts on palliative care from a social studies' perspective feature scant analysis of social work's contribution (Clark 1993; Clark *et al.* 1997; Sheldon 1997). This includes work where the focus is on how social divisions permeate the experience of dying and bereavement (Field *et al.* 1997).

The one current UK text which does take social work's role in palliative care as its remit is Oliviere *et al.*'s *Good Practices in Palliative Care* (1998). Concentrating on hospice-based or linked initiatives, it provides an excellent guide to the diverse range of practice within the discipline of social work currently undertaken under the umbrella of palliative care. This includes detailed work with children facing bereavement, efforts to build patients' participation in the shaping of care programmes at an AIDS palliative care unit, and outreach work to nursing homes. It also highlights how groupwork can enrich social work. The importance of research informing practice is acknowledged, as is the principle that 'the ill person and families [are] the best guides to practice' (Oliviere *et al.* 1998: 1). But – with the exception of the account of BACUP, the cancer information service – the absence of independent, systematic research findings means that the accounts labour under the constraint of being professional social workers' views of their own performance. Consequently they constitute a ground-breaking survey in terms of putting such efforts 'on the map', but do not provide independently validated evidence on the benefits or otherwise of such work to service users.

In this context it is also important to note how professional social workers generally are organised in relation to palliative care. Their engagement can be placed under two headings. First, there is the pro-vision – by voluntary sector social workers, for the most part – of an intensive (mostly hospice-linked) service to a relatively small number of the total population with life-threatening illness (National Council for Hospice and Specialist Palliative Care Services (NCHSPCS) 1998). Second, local authority social workers are engaged in assess-ment and provision for community care services, highly relevant to the needs of the whole population concerned, but without an explicit focus on palliative care.

The current scene is exemplified in the following comments from a planning officer in a major urban social services department, inter-viewed by one of the authors:

> The social services would bar you from involvement in palliative care if you were an area team fieldworker. It's care management as-sessment only ... What I would call the true palliative care model – long-term contact, counselling, dealing with the terminal nature of the illness, a range of interventions – is only carried out by voluntary sector social workers (hospice-based); specialist hospital social workers externally funded and off the 'duty' system, e.g. in liver or kidney specialist posts; and HIV specialist workers funded through Department of Health and Trust money.
>
> (Personal communication 1998)

One of the consequences of this situation is that systematic evidence explicitly addressing the outcomes of local authority social services fieldworkers' input to palliative care in the UK is virtually non-existent. Therefore to build a picture of the significance of profes-sional social work's contribution to the experience of life-threatening illness as a whole, evidence has to be gleaned from studies focusing on feedback on symptom control and the requirements for home care, studies of residential care settings, and general studies of hospital-based palliative care.

Service users' evidence marginalised

Even where systematic studies in palliative care have been carried out, most have not drawn on direct feedback from service users/patients themselves but have used those closest to them or their informal or professional carers as proxies (Higginson 1993; Sheldon 1997). The case for not involving service users/patients directly has centred on the unreliability of their contribution in extreme ill health and the intrusiveness of research interventions (Higginson 1993). However, there is evidence that dying patients do wish to participate in research to help others (Mor *et al.* 1988, quoted in Higginson 1993: 41; McLeod forthcoming). Moreover no close correlation has been found between the views of these patients and those close to them: 'At the moment, we can tell only a little about what a person thinks (or thought) from their family member's assessment' (Higginson 1993: 4).

THE ABSENCE OF COMPREHENSIVE PROVISION

While the evidence on the benefits of palliative care is problematic, what is apparent is that assistance with physical, psychological and social requirements is far from comprehensive, creating inequalities between those who receive it and those who do not. One aspect of this, which provides a context for subsequent discussion, is the range of locations in which people die and where they live in the year before their death. Only 7 per cent of deaths occur in hospices, compared to 12 per cent in nursing or residential homes, 24 per cent at home and 56 per cent in hospitals (Field and James 1993). A common pattern is that, while most people in Britain die in institutions, most of the last year of life is spent at home (Addington-Hall and McCarthy 1995; Clark *et al.* 1997). Surveying differences in pain relief and symptom control across these settings produces a harrowing picture.

Dying from cancer

The vast majority, approximately 96 per cent, of patients who receive hospice, in-patient, day centre or home care have cancer (Addington-Hall 1998). Substantial populations of terminally ill cancer patients die either in a hospice or specialist palliative care unit (17.5 per cent) or under the care of a domiciliary palliative care team (39 per cent) (Eve *et al.* quoted in Addington-Hall 1998: 12). Nevertheless, people who are dying from cancer still feature prom-inently amongst those lacking adequate resources and care, including social work care, while terminally ill.

Pain relief

Addington-Hall and McCarthy (1995: 295), in a study based on 2,074 cancer deaths across twenty health districts, found from reports by close family members/caregivers that 47 per cent of those being treated by GPs and 35 per cent of hospital patients had received treatment 'only partially controlling pain *if at all*' (our emphasis). In the last week of their lives, 61 per cent had been in a very distressing state of pain. Sykes *et al.* (1992), interviewing a sample of 106 carers in Pontefract, found one-third felt pain control had been inadequate in the deceased's experience. The degree of suffering this can represent in daily life is conveyed by this account of getting out of bed by a respondent with bone metastases, from a study by one of the authors (McLeod forthcoming):

> 'One day I just could not get out of bed; I screamed and I cried because I was in the middle of the bed, I'd got to get to the edge of the bed before I could get myself up. My husband couldn't get me out, I couldn't get out, we couldn't do it together and I said "Just leave me," I said, "get me one of my painkillers and I'll just have to be here until it works," and it took me about an hour after that before the pain had gone sufficiently to allow me to get out of bed.'

Control of other symptoms

A range of other symptoms experienced in the last year of life by over half Addington-Hall and McCarthy's sample included 'loss of appetite, constipation, dry mouth or thirst, vomiting or nausea and breathlessness' (1995: 299). Just over a third of the sample had experienced loss of bladder or bowel control and more than 60 per cent of these had found this very distressing. Such symptoms had also not been effectively controlled for a substantial proportion of people, with about one-third who suffered from nausea or vomiting finding that treatment had relieved it 'a little or not at all' (1995: 300).

Psychosocial care

Alongside the absence of effective treatment of physical symptoms, a number of studies have revealed a worrying situation where a range of psychosocial requirements is not being met. A fundamental requirement for organising personal affairs is accurate and full information about the conditions from which people are suffering. Addington-Hall and McCarthy (1995) reported that half their respondents had been unable to get all the information they had needed concerning the patients' illnesses. Hall *et al.* (1996) described how over half their sample of women with advanced breast cancer had found information given about the illness by specialists was confusing. Again, in Addington-Hall and McCarthy's (1995) study, a large proportion of the people who had died (25 per cent) had not been thought to know their death was imminent. While such important issues could be seen as primarily the responsibility of health care staff to address, others clearly lay within social work's ambit.

Addington-Hall and McCarthy (1995) found that social services provision had been targeted on people who were living on their own. Approximately 50 per cent had had a home help and 25 per cent meals on wheels. However, approximately 40 per cent of these service users were reported to have needed more help with shopping, cooking and cleaning. Sykes *et al.* (1992) found that 58 per cent of patients in their locality-based study had not applied for any financial benefits, despite all being eligible.

Consistent with the picture of health care at home evident in earlier chapters, in most cases (81 per cent) it was relatives who bore the brunt of caring (Addington-Hall and McCarthy 1995). While most had found this rewarding, nearly 40 per cent had seen their daily lives severely restricted by the demands it made on them. Moreover, about a third of carers described themselves as having health problems of their own which had made it difficult to provide the care required.

Given the range of demands which people who are experiencing life-threatening illness (and their supporters) are grappling with, it is also not surprising that a substantial proportion are suffering emotionally. Nevertheless, surveys suggest that many are left unsupported by health and social care services. Hall *et al.* (1996) found that although half of their sample of women with advanced breast cancer were experiencing extremes of anxiety and/or depression, nearly 80 per cent had received no psychological support, either directly or by being referred on. In Addington-Hall and McCarthy's study (1995: 303) about two-thirds of the deceased were described as having 'felt low at some point in their last year of life', but counselling was not on record as a feature of social services' department input.

Dying from other life-threatening disease

There is mounting evidence that lack of recognition of the life-threatening nature of other diseases obscures the extent to which people dying from them may experience profoundly distressing symptoms and consequently as great a need as cancer patients for medical and psychosocial care. In the case of heart disease, Gibbs *et al.* (1998: 961), drawing on the only study to date which has investigated symptoms experienced in terminal heart disease, have reported that 'in addition to dyspnoea [breathing difficulties], pain, nausea, constipation and low mood were common ... At least one in six had symptoms as severe as those in-patients with cancer managed in hospices or by palliative care services.' A quarter of the respondents had spoken of wanting to die sooner. This wish was associated with older age (over 75 years) and having a greater number of very distressing symptoms (McCarthy *et al.* 1997).

A similar picture emerges from Skilbeck *et al.*'s (1997) study of people dying from chronic obstructive airways disease (COAD). They found that those concerned expressed a range of extremely distressing physical symptoms: as many as 95 per cent suffered extreme breathlessness, but pain, thirst and fatigue were also common. Many reported that they could not even 'lift a bag of sugar' (Skilbeck *et al.* 1997: 101). High levels of psychological distress, anxiety, irritability and depression were also described, alongside social isolation, with most being housebound.

In both conditions there was a dearth of support from health and social services. Substantial numbers of those affected had been unable to get enough information about the illness and its progression. Little or no relief of symptoms was reported in over a quarter of those dying from heart disease (McCarthy *et al.* 1997). Those with end-stage COAD found hospital care comprehensive but back in the community their experience of care was fragmented and *ad hoc* (Skilbeck *et al.* 1997: 105). Key aspects of social support were also lacking. In the case of people with COAD, help with accessing benefits, aids and adaptations, and additional support with the emotional demands they faced was in fact forthcoming where they had contact with specialist health visitors and nurses, but this only happened in 11 per cent of cases.

The state of provision

Despite better provision and recognition in the case of people with cancer, the preceding discussion bears out the truth of Addington-Hall's statement concerning all life-threatening illness: 'Existing health and social services are not fully meeting the needs of patients living with life-threatening diseases and their families, for physical, psychosocial ... care' (1998: 16).

SOCIAL DIVISIONS, ACCESS AND THE EXPERIENCE OF PALLIATIVE CARE

The absence of resources and care described above should be recognised as a disablist situation preventing those with life-threatening illness from gaining what should be theirs by right: access to the best quality of life available.

Pre-existing social divisions are also highly significant in shaping patients' and supporters' chances of obtaining resources and palliative care services which do exist, and their experience of any palliative care services received, including professional social work. We highlight, in turn, key dimensions that are implicated – relative poverty, ageism, racism, sexism, heterosexism and disablism. It will also become apparent that these interact with each other to compound the problems faced by those who are dying.

The negative impact of social disadvantage on the well-being of those with life-threatening illness, the association of this with an increased likelihood of entry into ill health, and a more indifferent experience of health care in the earlier stages of illness constitute a triple assault on people's welfare.

The impact of relative poverty

Relative poverty is significantly associated with where patients die, with well-being in the course of dying and with the chances of a lengthier lifespan once terminally ill. Most cancer patients have been shown to prefer to have the chance of dying at home (Townsend *et al.* 1990). However, Higginson *et al.* (1994) found that the opportunity to do so is associated with income level. Their five-year study of place of death revealed a significant – eightfold – difference between the high proportion of cancer deaths which took place at home in the most affluent electoral wards as compared with the least affluent.

As our previous discussion revealed, the chances of well-being in the course of dying are marred by lack of access to palliative care services. Grande *et al.*'s (1998) review of studies of home care services has shown that cancer patients in higher socio-economic groups are not only more likely to die at home but are also more likely to access home care. Precisely how socio-economic status produces this situation is not clear; the most relevant factor may be area of residence, income, or occupation. As Grande *et al.* point out, it is crucial to disentangle which social processes are involved in order to ensure that any expansion of services improves access for less advantaged groups, rather than exacerbating existing inequalities in uptake. The scandalous situation remains in Britain at present that people who are terminally ill, although exempt from the waiting period to access attendance allowance and disability living allowance (Department of Social Security 1997a and 1997b), are nevertheless still means-tested (and so may be charged) for social care provided through social services.

The importance of removing financial barriers to the provision of such care is further highlighted by studies which have shown that referral to home care is associated with longer periods of survival following diagnosis (Gray *et al.* 1987; McCusker and Stoddard 1987 cited in Grande *et al.* 1998: 574).

Detailed accounts of living with terminal illness in relative poverty also illustrate how the negative effects of inadequate income permeate all corners of life. In Bourgeois's study of young men with AIDS on below average income, she found that adequate money 'for necessities ... for emergencies ... and for extras' constituted major worries on a daily basis, with 'enough money for necessities' representing the young men's chief concern, even superseding 'health' (1998: 78). In their account of social class differences in the last year of life, Seale and Cartwright (1994) reported that, despite being older at the point of death, middle-class subjects had not had more symptoms and attendant restrictions nor a worse quality of life than working-class subjects. Income did seem to have made a difference: 43 per cent of middle-class subjects, but only 30 per cent of working-class, were described as having had a good quality of life in the year before death, and money problems had featured in this. Twice as many working-class subjects – 15 per cent compared to 7 per cent – had found the cost a barrier to keeping their home adequately heated. Again, twice as many working-class subjects – 32 per cent compared to 16 per cent – were described as having needed more financial help. This also reflected benefits levels too low to be relied on to meet financial requirements, with 40 per cent of those on income support considered to have been in this situation while dying.

Ageism

The experience of being terminally ill in relative poverty shades into discussion of older people's experience in terminal illness. This is because the majority of those in this condition are over 65 and have levels of income which amount to living in relative poverty (Independent Inquiry 1998). Interacting with ageist tolerance of widespread poverty amongst older people, a further spectrum of ageist assumptions and conditions characterises older people's experience of terminal illness. In two seminal articles, Harris (1990) and Cowley (1990) highlighted evidence that older people constitute 'an underclass of dying people ... the disadvantaged dying' (Harris 1990: 29). This is partly because of the concentration of palliative care resources on those dying of cancer, rather than on the wider range of chronic illness older people experience. It is also in part because of the shortfall in resourcing health and social care services to meet older people's actual requirements, and because of ageist assumptions which have 'attributed such symptoms to age rather than to any underlying disease' (Cowley 1990: 30) and hence resulted in their neglect.

Age has been found to be a significant factor both in accessing home care and in hospice admissions. Older people are less likely to be referred for home care (Grande *et al.* 1998). Those aged over 85 are significantly less likely to be admitted to hospice care (Addington-Hall *et al.* 1998). This is despite the greater likelihood of their living alone, having a greater number of additional health problems and a greater degree of physical impairment (Victor 1991).

Dying alone

Older people are also more likely to die alone. Seale and Cartwright found that people who lived alone 'were most likely to die alone: 36 per cent did so, as opposed to 20 per cent of others living in private households' (1994: 72). That older women have fewer surviving male partners may constitute one dimension of this situation. It may also be the case that death occurs suddenly. Nevertheless, the associations between relative poverty, ageist discrimination and social isolation are so strong (Wilkinson 1996b; Arber and Ginn 1991) that their imprint would seem to be present here.

This is borne out in Howes' (1997) account of 'found deaths' amongst older people in five London coroners' districts. Such deaths referred to those over 60 who lived alone and were found dead at home with no one else present, and constituted between 20 to 25 per cent of all home deaths of older people in the area. In approximately 60 per cent of cases there was a record of chronic health problems, most commonly 'heart disease, high blood-pressure, arthritis and respiratory disease' and for those for whom such information was available, a further 'recent deterioration in state of health' had been noted in 20 per cent of cases (Howes 1997: 18). The bleak social conditions reflected in these statistics are represented in the following brief accounts:

> [Mr B] aged 72 years was found dead in his flat in Holloway in February 1995 after a local shopkeeper realised that he had not seem him for over a month. Mr B used to visit the shop every day to buy cigarettes and bread.
>
> (1997: 1)

> 70-year-old man. Cause of death – carcinoma of the lung. The cancer had recently spread to the brain; receiving regular treatment at St Bartholomew's Hospital, though he had not been seen by his GP for about two months. No mention of family or friends.
>
> (1997: 18)

> 88-year-old man. Cause of death – bronchial pneumonia. Deaf. Appeared to have no means of heating in the house. Seen by doctor ten days before death. Was a very independent man who refused medical and social services help. Found by neighbour on a visit.
>
> (1997: 20)

In hospital

In the context of the overstretched, under-resourced hospital care, underfunded home care and shortcomings in residential care discussed in earlier chapters and below, older people's experience of hospitalisation when terminally ill is problematic. Most people dying in hospital from a terminal illness are older people (Seale and Cartwright 1994). The current government, identifying palliative care in hospitals as a key target for development, acknowledges that all is far from well and that shortages of resources are implicated.

> For those dying in hospital too often the care and support for them and their families is not as good as it should be. With staff under enormous pressure, it can sometimes happen that bad news is broken insensitively, families are given inadequate information and support and dying patients receive poorer care than they deserve.
>
> (NHS Executive 1998: 2)

Specialist palliative care teams available to provide treatment and advice and training for other colleagues are now present in most hospitals, though comprehensive evidence of the extent of their impact on hospital practice is not yet available (Glickman 1996). The pattern of hospital admission in the last year of life is of short stays. This might not be worrying *per se*, but Seale and Cartwright (1994) found that in approximately 25 per cent of cases those close to the deceased felt discharge from hospital in the year prior to death had been premature and accompanied by inadequate provision of home care services. Admission to hospital in the last year of life is significantly lower for older people living in residential or nursing home care than from home (Seale and Cartwright 1994), although sadly the care received during the course of terminal illness in residential and nursing home settings cannot be relied upon to be of high quality.

Residential and nursing home care

As Field and James (1993: 17) have argued, evidence on the conditions in which older people are dying in residential and nursing home care is 'sparse and sometimes contradictory'. Nevertheless, three worrying features are discernible. First, the population concerned is for the most part a very vulnerable, socially isolated group. Seale and Cartwright (1994) found that two-thirds were aged over 85. Only one in twelve of those admitted during the last year of life – the inference being that they were to die in residential care – was thought to have 'a good quality of life', compared to about half of those admitted earlier. A poor state of health was prevalent, with constipation, mental confusion, incontinence, hearing and visual impairment being rife (Seale and Cartwright 1994). This was compounded by the desolate nature of older people's existence. Cartwright (1991) found that one in five of those residents who spent the whole of the last year of their lives in residential or nursing home care had either no visitors, or fewer than one a month.

Second, despite such profound needs, a good quality of care is not guaranteed. Gibbs (1995) found, for example, that pain relief available in nursing homes was inferior even to that in hospitals. Staff in nursing homes practised less advanced techniques, as a result of fewer opportunities for training, and specialist palliative care back-up was absent. Like Seale and Cartwright (1994), she also found that GP care was of variable quality, marked, in some cases, by a reluctance to visit (1995). Third, there is evidence that the event of a resident's death in nursing and residential homes still tends to be marginalised through various procedural manoeuvres (Komaromy 1998), instead of cultures being created to integrate, in the interests of all residents, this event which is 'likely to touch closely on their own situation' (Field and James 1993: 20).

A gendered experience of dying

This account of ageism affecting the experience of dying should also be read as one patterned by gender – for women predominate in the population of those aged over 85, in relative poverty, with multiple health problems and dying in institutional care (Grande *et al.* 1998; Victor 1991).

Women's experience of terminal illness across the age range is in fact marked by gendered disadvantage. Croft (1996) has produced a moving account of issues raised by women she has worked with as a hospice social worker. She identifies among women a tendency, ingrained through socialisation, to place their responsibility to care for others first, to the detriment of their own interests, including their health and well-being. 'As it is in life, so it seems to be in death. Central to most women who are dying is their internalisation of responsibility and concern' (1996: 77). One example she cites is Caroline, aged 68, who:

> was ill in bed with persistent vomiting. She looked pale and thin and her family were very worried. As soon as her 31-year-old daughter had gone out of the room Caroline said to me 'It's Sally I'm worried for ... how she is going to manage?'

> (Croft 1996: 77)

Of course it also remains the case that women either as lone parents or within partnerships are the prime carers of children and of other adults – a powerful force for shaping such attitudes.

Both Croft's (1996) account and the experiences of HIV-positive women (Positively Women 1994) also testify to how frequently women's experience of being gravely ill is marked by having to cope with the stringencies of relative poverty.

Racist tendencies

While awareness of how sexism informs the experience of terminal illness may be at a very early stage of development, two major concerns regarding racist tendencies are already apparent: that members of minority ethnic groups are disadvantaged in gaining access to palliative care, and that they face institutionalised racism when they do so. For example, the NCHSPCS (1995a) found that hospice in-patient and home care services lacked well-worked-out strategies to facilitate access by members of minority ethnic groups. There was an absence of translated information; members of minority ethnic groups were unaware of entitlement to services; GPs failed to refer when appropriate; and the Christian ethos of many hospices acted as a deterrent.

Attempts to address such problems have been made by producing translated information (Oliviere et al. 1998), appointing link workers to disseminate information and encourage appropriate referral (McLees 1996) and the development of a more multi-faith approach (Oliviere et al. 1998). Steps have been taken in some places to meet dietary requirements, provide interpreting services and help staff to be informed about and respond to diverse cultural requirements and rituals concerning impending death and bereavement (Oliviere et al. 1998).

Two criticisms of such initiatives have been raised, however. Both emphasise that simplistic organisational 'fixes' of complex issues run the risk of being racist themselves. First, Gunaratnam (1997 and 1998) has emphasised that existing multicultural models need to be changed. Her research has shown that workers in palliative care can confine themselves to a series of 'multicultural checklist' responses, as opposed to engaging with the intricacies of the emotional needs of members of minority ethnic groups in a more profound way. Through limiting themselves to this approach, consideration of how racism may be affecting working relations with service users can be sidestepped.

Second, Haworth *et al.*'s (1997) study of interpreting services in palliative care in an NHS trust emphasises the importance of sufficient investment in the development of services to combat racism. They found that interpreters lacked experience and knowledge of palliative care services, and also training in the issues raised by situations of terminal illness. Haworth *et al.* recommended not only the urgency of developing 'information, training and support which interpreters need to act effectively', but also that palliative care workers should invest time and effort 'to deepen mutual understanding of roles' (1997: 77).

Gay and lesbian experience

In the UK in the 1980s, as AIDS came to be perceived as a general threat to the population, anti-gay prejudice was amplified by government and media endorsement. In its most extreme form this was epitomised in the Conservative Family Campaign's call for 'the re-criminalisation of homosexuality and the isolation of the infected' (Alcorn *et al.* 1997a: 12). Such homophobic responses are now less strident, while initiatives emanating from the gay community, as we shall see below, are at the forefront of progressive developments in palliative care. Nevertheless, the organisation and provision of palliative care continues to be marked by institutionalised heterosexist discrimination. First, across palliative care as a whole, as opposed to gay men's health initiatives, the indications are that lesbian and gay rights and requirements are not uniformly recognised. This is reflected in their absence as an 'across the board' issue, from major policy documents concerning the expansion of palliative care (see Expert Advisory Group on Cancer 1995; NCHSPCS 1998).

Second, AIDS treatment itself is also marginalised. Over two-thirds of those who have been diagnosed with AIDS in Britain have been gay men (Alcorn *et al.* 1997b: 67). Provision for medical and social care is now established through the NHS and social services (Alcorn *et al.* 1997a). However, Small (1997) has shown that organisationally, palliative care for people with AIDS occupies a very vulnerable position. Government policy requires palliative care and treatment in AIDS to be integrated in provision for palliative care generally (NHS Executive 1996). Yet the situation remains one of concentration in specialist HIV/AIDS services (Eve *et al.* 1997 quoted in Addington-Hall 1998: 12). This leaves provision for palliative care in AIDS very exposed to cutbacks in public funding, while, contrary to popular belief, AIDS charities are less well supported by public giving than, for example, those concerned with cancer (Small 1997).

The advent of triple combination therapy underwritten by significant improvements in monitoring indications of disease progression has dramatically slowed the death rate from AIDS and progression to AIDS (Carne 1998; Gottlieb 1998). The movement of public funding away from specialist palliative care to underwrite such drug treatment (Parsons 1997) at first sight may therefore seem logical. However, the numbers infected with HIV and the need for palliative care to meet the formidable emotional, social and physical demands of AIDS (Bourgeois 1998) will continue to rise (Small 1997). This is the context in which the dismemberment of existing specialist AIDS palliative care facilities in the voluntary sector is taking place (London Lighthouse 1998).

Third, without AIDS as a focal point for activism (Richardson 1994), lesbian women's requirements in palliative care continue to go relatively unseen compared to those of gay men. The way in which heterosexist assumptions permeate all corners of institutional engagement with lesbian women's lives in the course of life-threatening illness is revealed in Croft's identification of the range of heterosexist assumptions that need challenging: 'about partners, families and children in support services, related problems of confidentiality and the possibility of exclusion from decision-making following the death of a partner' (1996: 86).

Disabling stigma

The disablist impact of stigma associated with illness, discussed in Chapter 4, is exemplified by two facets of palliative care. First, as Alcorn *et al.* (1997a: 23) have noted, although public attitudes in the UK have shifted, 'bigoted responses to people with HIV and AIDS have persisted throughout the epidemic, fanned by the tabloid press'. The majority of women with HIV/AIDS reported in Positively Women's survey (1994) had experienced stigma in the form of discriminatory treatment from health care workers, family and friends. This had undermined their chances of obtaining much-needed support with the emotional, social, material and care requirements they now faced.

Second, one of the aims of the hospice movement is that the in-patient care they provide should facilitate the continued integration into social life of people who are terminally ill, through recognising and responding to their psychosocial needs (see Saunders 1996; Sheldon 1997). Nevertheless, hospice in-patient care may in practice fulfil a different function in society. From a hospice-based observational study, Lawton (1998) has argued that admission to a hospice for the control of intractable symptoms constitutes a process of social exclusion. Her study revealed that such admissions predominantly concerned people whose physical integrity was beginning to disintegrate: 'Amongst the most common [reasons for admission] were incontinence of urine and faeces, uncontrolled vomiting (including faecal vomit), fungating tumours ... and weeping limbs which resulted from the development of gross oedema in the patient's legs and/or arms' (1998: 128). Lawton suggests that 'hiding away' people in this state in hospices or hospitals serves to perpetuate the disablist myth that the 'normal' state of our bodies – indissoluble from our personal identity – is that of being physically intact.

RESPONSES TO INEQUALITY IN LIFE-THREATENING ILLNESS

We have shown that the experience of life-threatening and terminal illness is characterised by the advances in treatment and care largely developed across the past thirty years, but also that evidence of progress is more equivocal than at first sight. Moreover, the provision of resources and care essential to well-being is far from comprehensive, creating a disablist situation. This is permeated by the interactive effects of social divisions, producing indefensible suffering on a wide scale. It is therefore crucial to assess the roles of government and social work in tackling these conditions. First, we examine salient features of government policy, then problematic facets of the current social work response. We conclude by identifying key aspects of contemporary activism which are attempting to challenge the discriminatory power relations which undermine a more equal chance of well-being when facing death.

THE GOVERNMENT'S RESPONSE

Some acknowledgement of key problems

To date, the current government has addressed problems in provision for people facing life-threatening illness in a series of policy pronouncements and measures. It has declared that care to promote physical and psychosocial well-being should be made available for 'all those who face life-threatening illnesses' (Addington-Hall 1998: 5) and has pinpointed two particularly daunting features of the experience of terminal illness: pain, and symptoms characterising the last few days of life (NHS Executive 1998; WPCGPC 1997; 1998). It has agreed that an equivalent standard of care should be 'integrated into the whole of NHS practice' (NHS Executive 1998: 2), to include both hospital and primary care.

Taken together with the general principle of tackling inequalities in access which runs through health policy generally (for example, in the objectives of Health Improvement Programmes and Primary Care Groups or PCGs) this should mean that tackling differential access to palliative care is automatically on the policy agenda. Since PCGs are envisaged as having a lead role in commissioning palliative care (Tebbit 1998) this should also focus attention on how multi-agency provisions for domiciliary palliative care are faring.

Absence of adequate measures for expansion of palliative care

Under the current government, equal state and charitable funding for voluntary sector hospice provision has not been reinstated (Clark 1998). However, provision for palliative care input at consultant level as integral to the development of cancer treatment centres (Expert Advisory Group on Cancer 1995) has been maintained. This, combined with the current government's commitment to improve NHS funding levels (see Chapter 5), means that palliative care does not face the bleakest scenario of funding being cut back, but at least four areas of concern remain.

First, no plans are discernible for the massive expansion of funding for health and social care in general, and palliative care provision in particular, which we have shown to be essential for adequate levels of palliative care. The minimum criteria for medical and nursing input put forward in a Department of Health working group on primary care in cancer are that primary care teams should have 24-hour access to specialist palliative care advice and admission to specialist palliative care, combined with 24-hour access to community nursing care (Tebbit 1998). The scale of increased funding required simply to meet the in-patient component of this proposal is reflected in Wilson *et al.*'s study (1995), which estimated that unmet need for in-patient and respite palliative care facilities for *non-cancer* patients in one health area, Thames Valley, alone was 66,000 bed days per year, an increase of two-thirds on the current provision of 40,000 bed days for cancer patients.

Second, the removal of means-testing for community care or nursing home/residential care input to palliative care is not yet on the government's agenda. Third, as discussed previously (see Chapter 5), the projected level of increase in hospital funding, incorporating increases in nurses' pay, seems unlikely to raise staffing levels to a degree that will make feasible any of the significant improvements in routine care and contact required to underpin the quality of palliative care available.

Finally, the government's blueprint for the development of palliative care does not bear the imprint of service user involvement, either in the planning and commissioning of care or in the organisation of research to determine need (Clark 1998). Collective representation of service users' interests in this field is not altogether in its infancy, however, as discussed below (pp 147–153), and, given the already well-developed models of collective representation in operation for disabled service users (Evans 1996; Evans and Fisher 1999), could certainly be boosted through government funding and recognition.

Beyond care and treatment

As our earlier discussion demonstrated, government policy is significant for life-threatening illness beyond the spheres of health and social care. For example, policies for equalising income across the population are as germane to life-threatening as to other serious illness: the spectre of relative poverty haunts the experience of dying. Underwriting a more equal chance of well-being while dying would require, at least, substantial improvements in pension levels, but also marked equalisation of income across the life course. As discussed in previous chapters, the government's approach to this has been tentative at best.

THE PROFESSIONAL ROLE OF SOCIAL WORK

The earlier discussion revealed a bleak scene concerning the outcomes of the lack of professional social work input overall in life-threatening illness, a picture of widespread failure to meet material, social, emotional and information requirements and of neglect in nursing home and residential care. Despite its commitment to addressing social disadvantage, the social work profession as a whole has also failed to raise public debate about the generally disadvantaged position of people with life-threatening illness and of particularly disadvantaged groups within this population. This situation is all the more disconcerting because such evidence as there is suggests that when interventions germane to social work do take place, service users benefit.

Practical services

Studies across several different sub-populations point to the provision of home care and of help with accessing benefits entitlements as being greatly valued. HIV-positive women reported a high degree of satisfaction with specialist HIV/AIDS social services workers, appreciating the practical and emotional support that they provided (Positively Women 1994). Practical services, such as cleaning, shopping and cooking, were identified by nearly all the women as making the difference between remaining at home and going into hospital. Warwick (1993), also reporting on the home care requirements of people who are HIV positive, found practical help accessed through social workers to be most highly valued. This included increased benefits and advice, home care and the co-ordination of services.

Support with emotional demands

There are indications that support with the emotional demands of facing death which, in principle, lie within social workers' repertoire is not only appreciated by service users but may also have positive outcomes (SSI 1993).

Heaven and Maguire's (1997) research bears out the importance of professional contact being structured so as to provide optimum chances for people to confide their worst fears. Their sample covered 87 patients with cancer who were estimated as having less than two months to live, and were assessed by nurses in the course of their work. It had been thought in advance that the patients would find it helpful to offload their concerns to the nurses, but in practice they simply tended to disclose physical symptoms. When the researcher contacted the same patients, employing approaches to facilitate disclosure such as signalling that the researcher was fully prepared for highly charged emotional issues to be conveyed, the patients described a far fuller range of anxieties. These included worries about their appearance, being a burden on those closest to them, the effects of loss of energy and fears for the future.

Littlewood (1992) found that carers who had lost a close family member particularly valued the continuation of emotional support from professionals whom they had got to know and had found supportive prior to the deceased's death. This endorses the potential value of hospice social workers' continued contact after bereavement, but also places a further question mark against the limitations on SSD fieldworkers' engagement with service users that are imposed by the rigidities of care management assessment. As the local authority planning officer already quoted put it: 'Pre-bereavement counselling is unheard of in area teams' (personal communication 1998).

Moving forward

The nature of the involvement of professional social work in the course of life-threatening illness, as discussed so far, reveals at least four prerequisites for its further development in service users' interests. First, the disadvantaged position of potential and actual service users who are grappling with life-threatening illness needs to be put on the generic agenda of discourse and practice. Too much is at stake, for them and for others close to them, for it to be assumed that this is an issue that can be contained by the efforts of a relatively small number of specialist social workers. The closer integration of local authority social services with NHS primary care may help here, but only to the extent that palliative care provision is made a priority. The indications are that this cannot be relied upon, given the competing demands on primary care and social services (Clark 1998).

Second, in support of the above, systematic evaluation is needed of both specialist and more wide-ranging social work input. This is to clarify social work's strengths in palliative care and also to obtain a fuller picture of problems attributable to its deficits across a wide range of settings – home, hospital, day care, nursing home and residential care.

Third, increased government funding of the types of services and interventions accessible in theory through social work input is essential. This is poignantly underscored by Clark *et al.*'s (1996) follow-up study of service users discharged from hospital. They found that the rationing of community care budgets meant that the basic amenity of being bathed could be withheld from service users even when they were terminally ill. The way in which a social worker caught in this web of inadequate resourcing struggled to do her best for the service user concerned, but against the odds, is graphically illustrated in the following extract:

> Although Mrs K had reached the cost ceiling of her care input and ... no more services could be supplied, she [the social worker] did in fact once manage to squeeze assistance with a bath out of the budget. Mrs K who was confined to her bedroom found this 'lovely and re-freshing'. The social worker felt this was important to Mrs K's quality of life, which she saw as 'limited', but she was unable to achieve this again before Mrs K died.
>
> (Clark *et al.* 1996: 36)

The remaining prerequisite for enabling professional social work to contribute more effectively to the provision of a more equal chance of well-being for people with life-threatening illness is a change in the power relations currently informing the availability and nature of care and resources.

SELF-HELP ACTIVISM

Running through our account is evidence that, despite the efforts of lay health workers and the dedication and hard work of the professionals involved, unjust, unnecessary suffering is occurring in the course of life-threatening illness. This constitutes a widespread abuse of human rights: the right to an equitable share of available material and social resources through to the end of your life, and to the best available care and treatment irrespective of your physical condition and social position.

This situation points to the centrality of the need for greater equality in the power relations affecting people with life-threatening disease. There is as yet no equivalent self-directed, unified and recognised social movement spanning life-threatening illness in parallel to the disability rights movement. However, a series of diverse initiatives is attempting to reformulate the inequitable power relations beyond and within palliative care. The linchpin of this activity is collective self-help activism engaged in tackling social inequalities with some professional support, including that of professional social workers. As such it has fundamental similarities with the model of social work for greater equity in health which has featured in our discussion of other dimensions of physical well-being. We now discuss salient features of such activism in the UK. These include:

- the identification of what is at stake as a question of rights
- incremental changes in power relations concerning treatment and care, comprising
  (a) equalising access to information
  (b) service user control over the organisation of treatment and care
  (c) service users having a central role in knowledge creation and research;
- collective action to tackle social disadvantage within the experience of life-threatening disease
- collective representation of the interests of people with life-threatening disease.

The influence of more general social movements such as gay rights and the women's movement pervades such initiatives, but they also reflect attempts to address social disadvantage within the population of those who are dying and consequently to tackle dimensions of social disadvantage which affect society as a whole.

An issue of civil rights

The notion of identifying the situation of people with life-threatening illness as a human rights issue is not novel. Mann (1991) has described how the conceptual leap was made by gay activists in the early days of HIV/AIDS treatment activism. Throwing off a passive patient role, which involved ceding the organisation and direction of treatment to professionals and acquiescing in governmental control of resources, they invoked instead the concept of human rights: non-discrimination, equality and justice, as principles which should inform their situation and treatment. These ideas have, however, remained largely confined within gay men's health work, rather than gaining wider currency through the whole population of people with life-threatening illness.

Incremental changes in power regarding treatment and care

A civil rights perspective may not generally characterise activism concerning life-threatening illness. However, a series of initiatives have produced incremental changes in the power relations governing treatment and care.

Equalising access to information and a new status for experiential knowledge

The disempowering effects on people with life-threatening illness of being left in a state of ignorance were illustrated earlier in this chapter (pp 130–31). A key factor in changing such a situation is equalising access to information about the disease processes concerned, about opportunities for treatment and care and the state of their availability and quality. Raising the status of experiential knowledge is also of central importance.

One example concerns the BACUP cancer information service founded by Vicky Clement-Jones, a doctor who herself had cancer and realised that people needed readier access to up-to-date scientific information, information about resources and access to knowledge based on first-hand experience (Clement-Jones 1985). A recent evaluation illustrates how BACUP is helping to meet a substantial need. Across a ten-day period, 1,044 callers rang. Information was the principle requirement identified in people with life-threatening illness, while support was the most frequently expressed concern of friends and relatives (Venn *et al.* 1996).

HIV/AIDS' information networks, developed primarily by gay activists, have also played a significant role in opening up means of obtaining 'reliable, up-to-date information in an accessible form' (Watney 1996: 197) about treatments and their consequences. This clearly remains of critical importance for people with AIDS, who face the demands of taking decisions on whether or not to press for, or follow, new treatments with major consequences for their continued well-being, in the context of health service rationing (Alcorn *et al.* 1997a).

A self-help initiative by Marie Nally concerning breast cancer promoted the equalisation of access to factual and experiential knowledge through what was then the relatively novel medium of the Internet. Nally set up and maintained a web site, originally to provide information on British cancer organisations, at that time in short supply on the net. However, she extended this to create a forum for debate and discussion, incorporating feedback sections for personal experiences and views, including those on recently published books and aspects of current campaigns. Some indication of the opportunities thereby opened up is provided by the fact that the web site averaged 2,500 'distinct hosts' per month, i.e. individuals taking material back to their own site (McLeod 1998: 23).

Greater user control of treatment and care

The development of service user control over the organisation of palliative treatment and care has been characterised by three types of initiative. First, through the efforts of people with life-threatening disease new organisations have been set up to address previously unmet requirements. The C4Ward initiative founded in the UK two years ago is the first UK network to develop self-help support groups specifically to meet the requirements of women with advanced breast cancer (Burch 1997). At its heart lay the recognition by Alison McCartney, its founder, who herself had advanced breast cancer, that self-help support groups following initial diagnosis could be unhelpful because of their focus on cure. She needed to draw on the experience of women in a similar position to herself: 'I longed to talk to someone who knew what it was like, someone who had 'been there' before me' (McCartney 1995: 2).

Secondly, in the self-help tradition, people with life-threatening illness have taken on the role of being 'key workers' for each other and are now recognised as such. This is reflected in the self-help support groups for hospice service users facilitated by hospice social workers (Oliviere *et al.* 1998). It is exemplified more comprehensively still in the work of Positively Women, which has grown from a small self-help group set up in 1987 by HIV-positive women to become a national charity with a resource centre in London providing information and a range of services including advice work, support groups and complementary therapies (Alcorn *et al.* 1997a; Positively Women 1994). Still embodying the principle of peer support as of crucial importance, direct support services are provided by HIV-positive women. As Positively Women has expanded, several women have begun to perceive a power shift in the organisation towards professional workers (1994). However, the benefits of the opportunities provided for engagement with other women with HIV or AIDS in the course of using services continue to come through very strongly in user feedback: "'If you say you've had a bad day they know what that can mean, instead of someone who's done a course in HIV and thinks they understand. I hate that"; "It got me in touch with other women with the same problem and this made my condition more bearable"' (Positively Women 1994: 49).

Third, through collective action, procedures have been devised and implemented which represent significant developments in rebalancing professional/lay power. Perhaps the most striking example of this is an initiative which emerged from gay HIV/AIDS activism concerning the exercise of medical power in end-stage disease. The development and dissemination of 'advanced directives' or 'living wills' (Terrence Higgins Trust 1998) represent a means whereby the individual concerned can complete written instructions as to whether or not, and in what forms, they give their consent to life-prolonging treatment once they have reached a stage where they may no longer be physically and psychologically able to take that decision. The means of nominating someone as proxy is also incorporated (Terrence Higgins Trust and Centre for Medical Law and Ethics 1994). Advanced directives are limited to being applied in the precise circumstances identified in the document, but they are binding in law, have the backing of the medical establishment (BMA and the Law Society 1995) and constitute an important means of retaining direction of treatment notwithstanding extremes of physical and cognitive impairment.

User-controlled research

A further dimension to reshaping the power relations that affect the rights of people with life-limiting illness concerns the governance of research to ensure that issues are framed with regard to these people's experience and that issues of inequity are not glossed over. As Clark (1998) has argued, user involvement is needed in the actual organisation of research, not just in providing more information.

The lesson from the disability rights and social work service user movements is that it is only as collective service user representation grows that legitimacy and funding to back user-controlled research builds up (Evans and Fisher 1999). It is also important to mention that, as reflected in the earlier part of this chapter, some medical and social scientists have had a distinguished record in revealing the existence of social exclusion and opening up the apparently reassuring state of palliative care provision to reveal harrowing suffering.

Nevertheless, three research strategies consonant with the development of a more user-controlled approach are worth highlighting. First, research tools can be tailored to the requirements of service users, so that even when terminally ill their engagement in the audit of quality of services is viable. For example, Rathbone *et al.* (1994) designed a questionnaire so as to be brief and easy to complete by terminally ill patients. Of the patients in their study, 62 per cent completed it within three weeks prior to their death and approximately 25 per cent within a week prior to death. Nearly 60 per cent of the patients concerned identified problems not picked up in the doctor/nurse assessment, mostly of a psychosocial nature.

Second, users can be directly involved in data-gathering. To undertake its survey of service users, Positively Women recruited and trained HIV-positive women. There was some evidence that interviewees identified more closely with interviewers as peers and that this led to fuller accounts on some key issues. A higher percentage of women acknowledged difficulties in practising safer sex than is usually found in surveys on this issue (Positively Women 1994).

Third, where collective representation of people with life-threatening illness does exist, then it can operate as an authoritative body regarding research questions. In the experience of one of the authors, for example, C4Ward forum gave detailed guidance on what research interventions would be sustainable, and therefore acceptable, by the women concerned.

Tackling social disadvantage within the experience of life-threatening illness

The potential for collective action that targets social disadvantage within life-threatening illness is illustrated in the outcome of a C4Ward initiative to target self-help support group resources at older women with advanced breast cancer. Feedback from the women concerned indicates that group companionship, access thereby to advice on benefits and services, plus free transport to facilitate participation, have all been valuable in breaking the hardships of social isolation and relative poverty (McLeod forthcoming).

Initiatives addressing relative poverty in life-threatening illness are not only significant within the context of palliative care, but also extend the reach of action on income equalisation and exemplify input from palliative care professionals who are supportive of greater equality. So, for example, the Association of Hospice Social Workers successfully campaigned on behalf of those who were terminally ill for the abolition of the statutory waiting period before qualification for disability living allowance and attendance allowance (Oliviere *et al.* 1998). A decade later the National Council for Hospice and Specialist Palliative Care Services has made representations to government to exempt people who are terminally ill from means testing for residential or community care (NCHSPCS 1995b).

Collective self-representation

As the earlier discussion has indicated, the most comprehensive efforts in the UK to extend the collective self-representation of the interests of people with life-threatening illness are gay HIV/AIDS initiatives. However, gay AIDS treatment activism remains circumscribed by powerful forces. As we have shown (see above, pp 140–1), state and voluntary sector specialist treatment facilities are vulnerable to changes in government priorities for funding. It could also be argued, as Allen *et al.* (1995) have done with reference to the USA, that incorporation into organising and providing forms of treatment and care early on has drained activist energies away from pressing for more comprehensive state-funded provision. And it cannot at present be said that HIV/AIDS networks either represent, or seek to represent, the interests of the wider population with life-threatening illness.

The question of collective service user representation has begun to surface in hospice-based social work and is a live issue among the Association of Hospice and Specialist Palliative Care Social Workers (1997and 1998). Croft (1998) has argued that this should shape not only individual practice, but service provision and policy development. With the support of hospice social workers and activists in the wider service user movement, a seminar is planned to provide for the beginnings of collective hospice service user representation (Firth 1998). It is hoped that this will not just offer the opportunity for service user feedback on services, but also constitute a means for service users to present their views on policy issues to representatives of leading organisations in hospice and palliative care (personal communication, Oliviere, School of Social Science, Middlesex University 1999).

CONCLUSION

Following the model of the disability rights movement, significant preliminary elements of collective self-organisation to progress the right to an equal chance of well-being in the course of life-threatening illness do now exist, although in a disparate, faltering and relatively early stage of development. With appropriate support, the population concerned has also begun to operate collectively as informed and expert agents in securing well-being.

The issue of disadvantage within this population has begun to be addressed, too. The number and scope of collective initiatives exerting leverage on the inequitable power relations that inform the experience of life-threatening illness is building up. As this happens the possibility of collaborating with existing pressure groups – such as the disability rights movement, the pensioners' movement and anti-poverty lobbies – increases. This in turn improves the chances of broader alliances coming into being to press for the more equitable distribution of resources and status across society to the very end of people's lives.

Chapter 7

Developing a political presence

INTRODUCTION: REDRESSING THE IMBALANCE OF POWER

In Chapters 3 to 6 we have presented examples of gains secured for lay health workers through social work practice within and outside professional social work agencies. These have focused on action at the local and/or inter-personal level. But it has been apparent throughout that countering the factors involved in creating and sustaining inequalities in health also requires intervention on a wider basis. For example, redressing the inequitable distribution of income and wealth, and changing policies which result in substantial levels of homelessness amongst young people or in the discharge of older people from hospital without adequate sources of practical and social support, require action at government level. Racism, resulting in institutionalised inequalities in access to health care services, or homophobia, resulting in unprovoked violence, cannot be adequately remedied by action solely on a local or inter-personal basis.

Moreover, structural inequalities in the social, environmental and economic order reflect globalised conditions which are addressed or maintained through pan-national political and economic systems. To give a direct example, air quality in Britain is determined not only by industrial and traffic emissions and other factors within the UK but by 'transboundary pollution from Europe' (DETR 1999), while the motor and oil industries operate on a global basis (DETR 1998b). Equally, industries with interests in promoting the commodification of health as a lifestyle choice or extending private capital involvement in health care, health insurance and new medical treatments and technologies increasingly operate transnationally (see Chapter 2).

Therefore, in this final chapter we consider how social work aiming to tackling inequalities in physical health can complement work at an individual or local level by exercising influence on these wider dimensions of unequal power relations. Bringing out the intricacy of the skills and the complexity of the power relations involved, we explore four central elements of a strategic approach to this objective:

- developing strategic alliances;
- evidence-based activism;
- integrating local and national action; and
- pressure politics.

We do so by drawing on indicative examples of action on three key issues, the significance of which for greater equality in health has been evident throughout our analysis: unhealthy environments, institutionalised discrimination in the healthcare system, and relative poverty.

In conclusion, we underscore the argument of the book as a whole.

DEVELOPING STRATEGIC ALLIANCES

Given the scale and weight of the embedded institutional and structural forces generating and reinforcing inequalities in physical health, strategic alliances to secure increased purchase on the issues involved are a necessity. Social work alone patently cannot transform poverty or end ageism, and social work is not alone in seeking greater equality in health. Opportunities exist to create or join existing coalitions of interest. Such alliances represent a departure from traditional notions of 'inter-professional' practice in three main ways:

- they embrace a substantially wider range of potential allies (including service users; McLeod 1995b);
- they are based on shared objectives in tackling health inequalities rather than on common professional interests (Bywaters 1986); and
- they look to develop national and international dimensions in analysing and addressing these objectives.

Combating unhealthy environments

The opportunities for and value of such alliances are exemplified in concerted action to prevent asthma attacks through countering environmental threats. Although uncertainty about diagnosis complicates the picture (Bytheway and Furth 1996), the number of adults recorded as seeing their doctor about asthma has trebled in the past twenty years, so that around one in twenty-five adults now has asthma. Rates are even higher in childhood, with one child in seven affected: 1.5 million children. Asthma causes about 100,000 hospital admissions each year, the loss of 17 million working days and, for children, can lead to substantial periods of absence from school coupled with the stigma and loss of fitness which comes from being unable to participate effectively in sport (National Asthma Campaign 1999).

The primary causes of asthma are still unclear, but environmental pollution, including traffic fumes, work-based pollutants and cigarette smoke, house dust mites, materials used to manufacture furniture, and damp and inadequately heated housing, are at least implicated in triggering symptoms amongst asthma sufferers (Dockery *et al.* 1993; National Asthma Campaign 1999; Schwartz *et al.* 1993). Environmental pollution is no respecter of national boundaries, but the impact of poor air quality does not fall equally across the UK. Factors linked to social class and income, such as the proximity of housing to 'dirty' industries and main traffic routes, especially those frequented by lorries and buses using diesel fuel (Phillimore and Moffatt 1994), are significant. As far as external sources of pollution are concerned, even relatively low levels of sulphur dioxide and particulates emitted by the diesel engines of lorries and buses have been shown to have an impact on health and to result in raised mortality, leading researchers to call for a further increase in minimum standards of air quality (Katsouyanni *et al.* 1997).

In Liverpool, where the ten years to 1996 saw a 100 per cent increase in admissions to the Children's Hospital, a 150 per cent increase in Accident and Emergency attendances and a 300 per cent increase in out-patient attendances, lay workers and professionals across many agencies have come together to create a comprehensive strategy for the management of respiratory disease. During the early 1990s residents in the Vauxhall and Granby districts of Liverpool, including people with asthma, and primary health care staff raised concerns about the extent of respiratory ill health experienced during periods of peak pollution levels. This concern coincided with that of members of the local Friends of the Earth (FOE) group who were interested in developing projects demonstrating that local communities could be involved in monitoring air quality to acceptable scientific standards of accuracy. Air quality monitoring tubes designed to measure pollution levels were installed in two localities by FOE (Gardner *et al.* 1996; Liverpool FOE and Vauxhall Health Forum 1993). Managed by local residents, including asthma suffers who also monitored and recorded their own health, and analysed by an accredited laboratory, these showed that while annual average levels were below guidelines, readings for individual months exceeded the European Union advice, even on occasion the EU limit. Proving that pollution levels fluctuated widely while regulations are based on annual averages was a significant element in the development of the strategic approach to asthma prevention and management being adopted on Merseyside; it also provided individuals with asthma with a new basis for discussion of their illness with their GPs (Gardner *et al.* 1996).

Academic epidemiologists in Liverpool University with an interest in promoting the WHO's Healthy Cities 2000 programme and public health doctors with responsibility for population health became involved. As a result, over a period of several years a broad coalition was formed between the parties, also incorporating the health authority and local authority, to secure preventive and remedial action on respiratory disease in general and asthma in particular (Liverpool Health Authority 1997). Alongside asthma management programmes, educational programmes targeting schools and public warnings of excessive levels of pollution, direct attempts have been made to reduce engine emissions through traffic calming measures and calls to close a main trunk road through to the docks used extensively by heavy lorries.

Local involvement was a necessary element lending legitimacy to professionals' development of the Healthy Cities 2000 programme. Equally legitimacy has been given to local action by national self-help activism through the National Asthma Campaign, by the international environmental movement, by the current government's promotion of measures to cut environmental pollution (DETR 1998c) and by global events such as the 'Earth Summits'. The European Union's recent Integrated Pollution Prevention and Control (IPPC) regulations also underscored local authorities' responsibilities for local air quality management (DETR 1998c).

Parallel alliances impacting on national policy and international policy to prevent the impact of deteriorating environmental conditions on asthma are also evident, involving both work-based and party political representation. The National Asthma Campaign has developed working relations with other potential sources of leverage, for example, by backing the TUC's (1999) 'Out Of Breath and Out of Work' survey focusing on workplace asthma. Via the TUC, the National Asthma Campaign has also gained access to influence government policy through the Trades Unions and Sustainable Development Advisory Committee, jointly chaired with the Environment Minister, Michael Meacher. This parallels Friends of the Earth's links with other environmental groups and party politicians to increase pressure for reducing traffic pollution by promoting private member legislation (FOE 1998).

The need for such coalitions is clear in the light of counter-action by the road lobby. At the local level in Liverpool, road hauliers successfully brought pressure on the local council to prevent the closure of the trunk road through Vauxhall called for by community and voluntary groups in alliance with professionals (FOE personal communication 1999). At the national level, the British Road Federation (BRF), incorporating not only the freight transport industry but a whole range of interest groups including the Society of Motor Manufacturers and Traders, the AA, the RAC and other commercial groups such as Boots and Tate and Lyle, campaigns continuously for extensions and improvements to the road infrastructure and resists measures to reduce and regulate traffic, using direct action tactics if necessary (BRF 1998). At the European level, for example, directives on traffic pollutants regulating heavy duty engines emerge from a 'collaborative research programme jointly undertaken by the European Commission, the European vehicle manufacturers and European Oil companies' (DETR 1998b: 2).

The leverage which the powerful road lobby can exert at local, national and international levels reinforces the need for strategic alliances which also bridge these dimensions. Despite the success of the road lobby in securing a measure of control over the issue by collaborative work on the 'inside' with governments and transgovernmental organisations, the lobby's adoption of rhetoric about environmental concerns and engagement with pollution reduction measures can be seen as a measure of the effectiveness of environmental pressure groups internationally. Meanwhile, locally based alliances, such as that in Liverpool, provide some opportunity for the 96 per cent of the poorest fifth of UK households who do not have a car to have some voice in debates about traffic pollution (FOE 1998).

Professional social workers wishing to act on socially constructed health inequalities should lift their gaze, not just to encompass concerted action across localities, but also to start linking locally-based action into strategic alliances with national and international campaigns.

EVIDENCE-BASED ACTIVISM

We have identified how securing independent access to information, for example about material resources or about particular forms of ill health and their treatments, is a significant source of leverage for *individuals* attempting to redress the imbalance of power in their encounters with professionals. Information, sometimes in the form of independently obtained research evidence, is also valuable in *collective* action for change.

Tackling institutionalised discrimination

Obtaining and deploying information has been a key element of Age Concern's anti-ageist campaign to extend access to routine breast cancer screening beyond the arbitrary cut-off age of 65. Through commissioning new research and collating, analysing and publicising existing evidence in the public domain, Age Concern's breast cancer screening campaign exposed how the majority of deaths from breast cancer, 63 per cent (Age Concern England 1996a), occur amongst women aged 65 or over. Yet this age group is excluded from being routinely invited to take part in the NHS breast cancer screening programme (McHugh 1996). Older women aged over 65 can request screening but, prior to the Age Concern campaign, relatively few did so, as not many were aware that it was their right. In 1993/4, only 0.4 per cent of women aged 65 or over were screened on request. In the same year the take-up rate by women aged 50–64 was approximately 72 per cent (Age Concern England 1996a). There is substantial evidence from major research trials abroad of equally high take-up rates among older women when routinely included. Moreover, these trials indicate that as many as 2,000 older women's lives could be saved every year in the UK if they were routinely invited for screening (McHugh 1996).

The Conservative government resisted Age Concern's call for a change of this blatantly ageist policy. It established three pilot projects, each to last three years, in which screening invitations were to be offered to women aged between 65 and 69 (McHugh 1996).

However, the following official statement bore the hallmarks of using research as a delaying tactic prompted by financial considerations:

> Baroness Cumberlege – Lords Oral Answers on the pilot projects: [Extending the screening programme to women aged over 65] is a very expensive process to introduce nation-wide. We do not know at the moment how many women would take up this opportunity. We do not know what the costs would be in terms of the detection of cancers.
>
> (Hansard col. 1575, 6 November 95)

The next stage in Age Concern's campaign was the dissemination of publicity about older women's right to request screening once every three years, partly in order to test the implied government argument that older women would not wish to take up screening opportunities (McHugh 1996). It drew on its network of local offices, workers and volunteers to target older women directly on this issue, making use of a specially devised information booklet (Age Concern England 1996b). Three significant outcomes resulted. First, the campaign demonstrated older women's interest in this issue by producing the largest uptake of printed information in the organisation's history: 400,000 copies of its booklet on breast cancer screening and older women's rights were picked up or distributed (personal communication, research officer, Age Concern 1997). Second, as a result there is not only anecdotal evidence (from the same source) coming in from branches of Age Concern of an increase in requests for screening, there is hard evidence of a significant increase. Once Age Concern's campaign was under way in 1996, the numbers of older women screened by request rose from 39,193 in 1994–5 to 57,535 in 1997 (Perham *et al.* 1998). Third, based explicitly on this evidence of increased interest attributed to the Age Concern campaign, the issue was brought to public and government attention again, through sympathetic MPs presenting a parliamentary early day motion (Perham *et al.* 1998).

The current government is sticking to the policy of its predecessor in maintaining that it will not reach a conclusion on any policy changes affecting older women's access to breast cancer screening until the final report on the pilot projects becomes available in April 2000 (personal communication, health policy officer, Age Concern England 1999). This is despite the evidence already available constituting a conclusive case for change. One pilot study has already reported interim results of a take-up rate averaging 75 per cent in women aged between 65 and 69, with a cancer detection rate of 8:1000 in women aged 65–67 and 17.4:1000 in women aged 68–69 (Rubin *et al.* 1998).

The fact that the extension of breast screening has not yet been secured does not negate the value of evidence-based activism. The evidence collated and collected by Age Concern provided the mechanism for creating and maintaining public attention towards this issue through Parliamentary contacts, while also raising awareness of age-based discrimination in the health service – and of their rights – for hundreds of thousands of older women. As with AIDS treatment activism (Watney 1996), a combination of challenging exclusively professional control of research and information, and taking head on any arguments for inactivity or delay based on supposed lack of evidence, creates some valuable leverage for change.

INTEGRATING LOCAL AND NATIONAL ACTION

A key element in both the previous examples was that action by a community of interest to challenge environmental conditions or structural inequalities also secured direct gains for the communities concerned. Better management of care for people with asthma was secured through collaborative action between sufferers, primary care staff and public health doctors. School staff were educated so that sickness absence fell and participation in beneficial physical activities like sport was increased. Pollution warnings through the local media are planned (FOE personal communication 1999). Through Age Concern's campaign, many more women have been screened and cancers have been detected. Wider action on the structural conditions influencing health inequalities does not have to be an alternative to local and individual action – they can, and should, complement each another.

Tackling poverty

Our third example, the work of the credit union movement, shares this feature of inter-dependence between local and national action to secure tangible, if incremental, health gains. As demonstrated in Chapter 3, credit unions (CUs) bring health benefits to individuals and neighbourhoods grappling with relative poverty by making available accessible, affordable savings, credit and associated financial services. In doing so, they challenge at a local level the monopoly of profit-driven enterprises over determining the provision or lack of financial services, while offering significant material benefits for CU members.

Involved mainly in local community-based projects, the credit union movement has now grown to a point where it comprises a national network, has a national representative body – the Association of British Credit Unions Ltd. (ABCUL) – and a share capital of over £100 million (HM Treasury 1998a). However, a survey of half the CUs in the country found that 62 per cent were open for six hours a week or less, a third for three hours or less. For 86 per cent, it was felt that volunteer burn-out was restricting their growth. Only 17 per cent had their own premises and the average locality-based membership was 200 (Jones 1999).

In order to exert even more effective leverage on microfinancing, local development alone is insufficient. CUs have recognised the need for a larger membership base, more diverse and efficient service provision, and legal changes that would enable them to access financial resources from each other or from the financial world beyond the movement (Conaty and Mayo 1997). They have argued for the creation of a special legal status of 'community development credit union' for CUs operating among populations with high levels of relative poverty. This designation would grant entitlement to complete relief from corporation tax and rates on property, and exemption for volunteers from loss of benefit on grounds of not being available for work. CUs also propose the continuation of substantial levels of public funding to preserve a community development role.

Recognising the significance of CUs in tackling an important contributory dimension to relative poverty, the government established a 'Taskforce' to examine how banks can help CUs to develop further (HM Treasury 1998a):

> Access to financial services to those on low incomes is crucial if we are to prevent social exclusion. What we want to see is more banks, helping more CUs, helping more people get access to savings and credit facilities.
>
> (Economic Affairs Secretary Patricia Hewitt quoted in HM Treasury News Release 22 September 1998: 2)

Despite the successful achievement of government backing, however, two major limitations are apparent in this development. First, there is the risk that the Taskforce will lead to the incorporation of CU activity by the profit-making sector. There is a powerful banking presence on it, with the chairperson and seven out of the twelve representatives coming from banks or building societies, as against three representatives from the CU movement (HM Treasury 1998b). The obvious possibility is of a banking 'takeover'. Indeed, some commentators advocate the incorporation of business practices and ideals as the key to future development. Jones (1999: 4), for example, argues that CU development agencies 'should promote an image of credit unions ... away from the "poor man's bank" and see them as community-owned financial institutions [with] business planning tools which enable credit unions to develop and own business plans which show self-sustainability within 3–4 years'. However, this may bring the second danger: dilution of the CU movement's traditional commitment to retain a focus on the needs of poverty-stricken members (Conaty and Mayo 1997). Devising public finance incentives to banks in the commercial sector to re-establish a presence in neighbourhoods with high levels of poverty would not, for example, guarantee the continued access to low interest rates, flexibility of repayment arrangements and reciprocal personal support which CUs currently provide.

The legitimacy of the CU movement's pressure on government to change the conditions under which CUs operate depended upon the success of local projects in demonstrating the need for local financial institutions in disadvantaged areas and the effectiveness of financial management services designed to be accessible to people on low incomes. However, without also securing gains at a wider level, the impact of CU activity locally will be constrained. The national focus currently provides members of the population living in relative poverty with some, albeit limited, means of representation in negotiations involving those governmental and commercial institutions routinely involved in servicing capitalist interests, a voice which would not otherwise be present.

Demonstrating the links between individual and community experience of disadvantage and discrimination and the wider forces which oppose, resist or undermine action for change is a major spin-off. The politicisation of apparently individual problems offers counter-evidence and counter-experience to the public, victim-blaming discourse which presents health-related problems as 'just' sickness or old age or reflecting a dependency culture of poverty. The wider political dimensions are made transparent to all concerned. It becomes clear that asthma is not just a matter of personal tragedy perhaps brought on by unhealthy lifestyles; that blatant discrimination affects older women's access to life-saving health care; and that, far from being just a matter of personal failing, the difficulties of managing money when living in poverty are compounded by decisions based on profit maximisation for shareholders rather than on customer interest.

PRESSURE POLITICS

Even if government is sympathetic to the significance of health inequalities, government policy lies at the confluence of competing pressures, including those antithetical to health such as the drive to consume and commodify health in the interests of capital (see Chapter 2). Therefore it is important to sustain pressure on central government to push forward measures to equalise health, and our examples provide evidence of four strategies which contribute to this.

Engaging with established networks

First, one of the benefits of creating strategic alliances is that individuals and professionals come into contact with campaigning pressure groups which have already developed networks of influence. Although single-issue campaigns at a local level can result in interest from, for example, party politicians or the media, pre-existing networks, developed over time, are likely to be more effective. Again there is an interconnection of interest between local and national action. This is reflected in the way in which the environmental lobby, as represented in the work of Friends of the Earth, has succeeded in inscribing action on environmental issues into party political programmes, not only in the UK, but internationally. Thereby, social work engagement with environmental issues – in the Liverpool example, through community action in specific localities – can feed into collective action which represents a powerful political force in its own right. As Hoff (1997) has argued, these strategic steps need to be read as 'social work skills' which enable social work as a profession to play its part in environmental action in the interests of well-being.

Using the media

Second, alliances between local activists and national networks can generate media interest which can help to keep issues before the government's and constituents' attention. For example, the Liverpool asthma campaign attracted the attention of BBC prime-time national radio (*You and Yours* 16 March 99). The programme in question emphasised the extent of the populations affected, including children, highlighted the importance of focusing on preventive measures and stressed the relevance of combating traffic pollution in this context.

Backing from local government

Third, single-issue initiatives and networks representing communities of interest can target and gain valuable support within mainstream political activity at local government level. Local government has been a major long-term supporter of the development of CUs, providing recognition, start-up funding and personnel (Jones 1999). While currently the focus is on central government action, it is impossible to conceive of this having emerged without the bedrock of local government commitment to CU development across the past two decades, which has been integral to anti-poverty strategies (Sedgwick-Jell 1996).

Marshalling public support

Finally, in all our examples, the initiatives concerned have aimed to secure government backing as essential to achieving their aims. The establishment of the Credit Union Taskforce, for all its limitations, could not have been achieved by the CU movement alone but required the support of government. However, in a symbiotic way such initiatives may also help government to progress its aims through marshalling public support, thereby conferring legitimacy on particular policy positions. For example, the populist ring to the following Party Conference statement on health and the environment by Joan Ruddock, MP, when Shadow Environmental Protection spokesperson, testifies to how the growth of public awareness of pollution as an issue resonates with politicians: 'At heart, the fate of the environment is about the health of the people' (Socialist Health Association 1996).

CONCLUSIONS: SOCIAL WORK, HEALTH AND EQUALITY

In this chapter, as throughout, we have demonstrated that it is of vital importance for social work to address inequalities in physical health This has significant implications for how practice is resourced, defined and organised and constitutes both a crucial new focus for practice and a critical outcome of practice.

Re-sourcing social work

An inequitable triple set of obstacles to physical well-being has been experienced by both individuals and populations featured in our account. These comprise: the association between relative poverty and the greater likelihood of ill health; greater financial hardship following the onset of ill health; and reduced chances of subsequently securing a sufficient level of income to maximise health. Compounding this unjust situation, social services departments' and voluntary-sector professional social work agencies' efforts to help have been revealed as consistently undermined by inadequate funding, which has led to inferior responses and services, both in the promotion of well-being and in the course of ill health. Meanwhile, self-help initiatives have frequently operated on short-term shoe-string funding.

The rhetoric of current government policy recognises the material basis of health inequalities. As preceding chapters have shown, some elements of the financial redistribution which is essential to equalise health have been set in train. Social work has also been 'set to work' to focus on the issue of tackling – albeit only in a local context – the socially constructed bases of health inequality. However, in the project of creating greater equality in health, social work services can only fully succeed if adequately funded and if they operate against the background of an effective government commitment to a substantially more equal distribution of income and wealth.

Re-mapping social work

The scope of practice

Our analysis highlights that lay efforts, for example, those of campaigners, advocates, advice workers and support group members, together with non-social work professionals such as credit union development workers and nurse counsellors, are central to people's welfare. It also indicates that against the considerable odds referred to above, valuable work in the interests of more equitable health chances and experience may be carried out by professional social workers from a formal social work organisational base.

In addition, the importance of developing the repertoire of social work practice in the interests of progressing more equitalbe chances of health has become apparent. For example, action research uncovered medicine's limitations in responding to older women's health screening requirements. Community profiling opened up how institutionalised racism could be countered in health and social care responses. Information activism employing some of the latest technology emerged as a critical self-help tool, as did reciprocal forms of counselling.

Moreover, as set out earlier in this chapter, developing practice on health inequalities enables common cause to be made with more widespread initiatives. Creating and feeding into nation-wide and transnational networks enhances the chances of sustaining pressure on governmental policy agendas to become more conducive to fair chances of health. Therefore this type of activity should also gain recognition as an essential, strategic dimension to practice if it is to maximise its impact on health inequalities.

Lay–professional power relations

Throughout our account one organisational development has been critical to the creation of more egalitarian health-providing forms of practice. This is the realignment of the hierarchical balance of power between social work professionals and lay health workers, so that it is more in lay workers' favour. This has characterised measures to open up readier access to primary resources for health maintenance: income, safe shelter, supportive human contact. It has been the springboard for making information on treatment and care and the means of redress for insufficient care more readily available. It has been the essential preliminary to combating disablist stigma and securing an active presence in research and policy formation. Lay collective self-help targeting social disadvantage in the interests of greater equity in health has been the driving force in this development. Whether taking the form of, for example, gay men's health activism, Women's Aid, or action on ME, they have represented the creation of campaigning and service provision initiatives in their own right. The key roles for sympathetic professionals have been collaboration and work to build a supportive infrastructure.

A new focus for social work

Inequality in physical health is an issue of social injustice. The incidence of ill health, the chances of safeguarding your own health and that of others close to you, the physical and emotional demands of ill health, the work of recovery and the rigours of life-threatening illness are all shaped by the interactive effects of social inequalities. If social work's commitment to social justice is to be fully reflected in practice, inequality in health must be placed on the social work agenda and remain there.

Tackling inequalities in physical health also cannot be compartmentalised, kept apart from addressing other dimensions to social inequality; for just as inequalities in health are themselves a product of multiple, interacting aspects of social inequality, so they in turn reinforce other elements to social inequality. Our focus on tackling inequalities in physical health therefore argues for, not against, the importance of making attention to other facets of social disadvantage a central feature of social work discourse, policy and practice.

A critical outcome of social work

Recognition of inequalities in physical health as an issue for social work exposes social work's own complicity in compounding such inequalities. We have given evidence of the neglect of anti-poverty strategies which could make a significant difference to health-damaging choices, for example the choice between heating and eating. We have described the narrow, bureaucratised, rationing routines imposed on social workers who knew that a fuller repertoire of practice would have diminished the suffering associated with severe ill health. We have shown the inadequate impact which formulaic approaches to anti-racist strategies have had on equalising provision in the course of life-threatening illness. Such uncomfortable truths constitute a powerful reason why tackling inequalities in health should become central to practice.

However, the critical argument in favour of social work addressing inequalities in health is that in its own right social work generally, not confined to health care settings, *can* contribute to greater equality across major dimensions of health experience. Through explicitly focusing on the problem of how to achieve greater equity in health and through tackling social inequalities, social work can contribute to more equal chances and experiences of health, particularly in relation to:

- health creation and maintenance;
- profound ill health at home;
- hospitalisation; and
- facing death.

This outcome of practice represents the reduction of unjust, unnecessary, physically embodied suffering. On these grounds such practice should be integral to any social work which is concerned to promote greater social equality.

Notes

Chapter 1

1 Throughout, the policy documents we refer to apply to England. We recognise that different legislation, organisational forms and nomenclature may apply in Northern Ireland, Scotland and Wales.

Chapter 4

2 'Long-standing limiting illness' is a term employed in General Household Surveys. We recognise that it fails to make clear what constitute the 'limiting' factors respondents are referring to – which will commonly be disablist social conditions – but it has the advantage of being self- rather than medically defined and does provide a point of comparison over time.

3 Information about the Barnardo's Sherwood Project was provided in an interview with the project manager, Pat Green, and from the Barnardo's project report.

4 Information about Cancerlink is drawn from booklets and other published materials produced by Cancerlink, 17 Britannia Street, London WC1X 9JN.

Chapter 6

5 There is no entirely satisfactory terminology here. 'Life-limiting illness' is both too vague and has disablist connotations. 'Terminal illness' is increasingly being used to describe the very last period of illness – end-stage disease, or the last few days of life (Working Party on Clinical Guidelines in Palliative Care 1998). There is also growing recognition of the experience of 'terminal illness' as being less discrete, i.e. that people may be receiving life-extending or possibly curative treatment alongside palliative care (Clark and Seymour 1998). The term 'life-threatening' may represent a brief but passing acute phase in an illness. However, it has the advantage of acknowledging a central feature of what previously was more generally referred to as terminal illness, that in the context of currently available treatment and the disease process itself, death in the near future is an unavoidable consequence. It is also a term in increasingly common usage (see Addington-Hall 1998).

6 Palliative care: as Clark and Seymour (1998: 86) have argued, this is a 'slippery

concept ... subject to ongoing debate and reformulation'. NHS policy documents and the NCHSPCS have argued for differentiation between the 'palliative care approach', integral to health care irrespective of the nature or stage of the illness in question; 'palliative interventions', those administered for the relief of symptoms by non-specialists such as anaesthetists; and 'specialist palliative care services', those involving a range of practitioners, including social workers, specialising in palliative care.

7   There are four chosen limitations to the discussion presented here:

(a) We recognise the central importance of bereavement in human experience, the significance for well-being of how it is responded to and the leading role of sensitive and imaginative work on the part of hospice-linked social workers in this respect (Oliviere *et al.* 1998). However, within the confines of this chapter we concentrate on practice concerning impending bereavement or anticipatory grief prior to death.

(b) Social work involvement in assisted suicide and voluntary euthanasia has begun to surface in social work discourse (see Ogden and Young 1998). We do not see either activity as necessarily antithetical to the interests of people who are dying; however, we recognise not only that this is a highly contentious issue, but that the means of ensuring that these activities are in the interests of those who are dying is acknowledged (even by those who are supportive of such approaches) to be at a very early stage of development (Oxenham and Boyd 1998). Consequently we focus instead on discussion of Advanced Directives as one means of tilting the balance of power in decision-making on forms of intervention near death, more towards patients themselves.

(c) We do not feel qualified to debate the spiritual dimensions of suffering or the spiritual consequences of intervention by professionals, but do consider the importance of avoiding Eurocentric assumptions concerning religious practices.

(d) Finally, though we acknowlege that thoughtful, painstaking, work has been and continues to be developed with children living with life-threatening illness (see, for example, Oliviere *et al.* 1998), and have no wish to marginalise younger people's and their parents' experience, this is not a focus of this chapter.

Bibliography

Action on Aftercare Consortium (1996) *Too Much Too Young: The Failure of Social Policy in Meeting the Needs of Care Leavers*, Ilford: Barnardo's.

Adams, S., Pill, R. and Jones, A. (1997) 'Medication, chronic illness and identity: the perspective of people with asthma', *Social Science and Medicine* 45(2): 189–201.

Addington-Hall, J., Altmann, D. and McCarthy, M. (1998) 'Which terminally ill cancer patients receive hospice in-patient care?' *Social Science and Medicine* 46(8): 1011–16.

Addington-Hall, J. (1998) *Reaching Out: Specialist Palliative Care for Adults with Non-malignant Diseases*, London: NCHSPCS and Scottish Partnership Agency for Palliative and Cancer Care (SPAPCC).

Addington-Hall, J. and McCarthy, M. (1995) 'Dying from cancer: results of a national population-based investigation', *Palliative Medicine* 9: 295–305.

Age Concern England (1996a) *Briefings: Breast Screening and Older Women – Statistics*, Ref. 1595, London: Age Concern England.

—— (1996b) *Breast Cancer Screening: Your Rights and What It Means for Women Aged 65 or Over*, London: Age Concern England.

Age Concern London (1995) *Hospital After Thought: Support for Older People Discharged from Hospital*, London: Age Concern London.

Ahmad, W.I.U. (ed.) (1993) *'Race' and Health in Contemporary Britain*, Buckingham: Open University Press.

Ahmad, W.I.U. and Atkin, K. (1996) 'Ethnicity and caring for a disabled child: the case of children with sickle cell or thalassaemia', *British Journal of Social Work* 26: 755–75.

Ahmad, W.I.U. and Walker, R. (1997) 'Asian older people: housing, health and access to services', *Ageing and Society* 17: 141–65.

Ahmedzai, S. and Biswas, B. (1993) 'The medicalisation of dying', in D. Clark (ed.) *The Future for Palliative Care*, Buckinghamshire: Open University Press.

Alcorn, K. (ed.) (1997) *National AIDS Manual*, London: NAM Publications.

Alcorn, K., Bennett, D., Gorna, R., King, E., Mortimer, J., Evans, B. and Barlow, D. (1997b) 'Overview of the UK epidemic', in K. Alcorn (ed.) *AIDS Reference Manual*, London: NAM Publications.

Alcorn, K., Gorna, R. and Scott, P. (1997a) 'The history of AIDS', in K. Alcorn (ed.) *AIDS Reference Manual*, London: NAM Publications.

Allard, A. and Dunn, M. (1997) *House Our Youth 2000: Access Denied*, London: NCH Action for Children.

Allen, S.M., Mor, V., Fleishman, J.A. and Piette, J.D. (1995) 'The organisational transformation of advocacy, growth and development of AIDS community-based organisations', *AIDS and Public Policy Journal* Spring 1995, 10(1): 48–59.

Anderson, I., Kemp, P. and Quilgars, D. (1993) *Single Homeless People*, London: Department of Employment.

Anderson, R. (1992) *The Aftermath of Stroke*, Cambridge: Cambridge University Press.

Anderson, R. and Bury, M. (eds) (1988) *Living with Chronic Illness*, London: Unwin Hyman.

Anionwu, E.N. (1993) 'Sickle cell and thalassaemia: community experiences and official response', in W.I.U. Ahmad (ed.) *'Race' and Health in Contemporary Britain*, Buckingham: Open University Press.

Annandale, E. (1998) *The Sociology of Health and Medicine*, Cambridge: Polity Press.

Arber, S. and Ginn, J. (eds) (1991) *Connecting Gender and Ageing*, Buckingham: Open University Press.

—— (1993) 'Gender and inequalities in health in later life', *Social Science and Medicine* 36(1): 33–46.

—— (1995) 'Gender differences in informal caring', *Health and Social Care in the Community* 3: 19–31.

Aronson, J. (1998) 'Lesbians giving and receiving care: stretching conceptualizations of caring and community', *Women's Studies International Forum* 21(5): 505–19.

Association of Community Health Councils for England and Wales (ACHCEW) (1996) *The Patients' Agenda?*, London: ACHCEW.

—— (1997) *Hungry in Hospital?*, London: ACHCEW.

Association of Hospice and Specialist Palliative Care Social Workers (AHSPCSW) (1997) *Committee News Bulletin* No. 5, October 1997: 1–2.

—— (1998) *Committee News Bulletin* No. 6, April 1998: 1–2.

Atkin, K. and Rollings, J. (1993) *Community Care in a Multi-racial Britain: A Critical Review of the Literature*, London: HMSO.

—— (1996) 'Looking after their own? Family care-giving among Asian and Afro-Caribbean communities', in W.I.U. Ahmad and K. Atkin (eds) *'Race' and Community Care*, Buckingham: Open University Press.

Audit Commission (1992) *Homeward Bound: A New Course for Community Health*, London: Audit Commission.

—— (1997) *The Coming of Age*, London: Audit Commission.

Badawi, M. and Biamonti, B. (1990) *Social Work Practice in Health Care*, London: Woodhead Faulkner.

Balloch, S. and Robertson, G. (1995) *Charging for Social Care*, London: National Institute for Social Work/Local Government Anti-Poverty Unit.

Barlow, J., Harrison, K. and Shaw, K. (1998) 'The experience of parenting in the context of juvenile chronic arthritis', *Clinical Child Psychology and Psychiatry* 3(3): 445–63.

Barnardo's (no date) *Doing Time. Families Living in Temporary Accommodation in London*, Ilford: Barnardo's.

Barnes, C. and Mercer, G. (1996) *Exploring the Divide: Illness and Disability*, Leeds: The Disability Press.

Barnes, M. and Shardlow, P. (1996) 'Identity crisis: mental health user groups and the "problem" of identity', in C. Barnes and G. Mercer (eds) (1996) *Exploring the Divide: Illness and Disability*, Leeds: The Disability Press.

Barrow, M. and Bachan, R. (1997) *The Real Cost of Poor Homes: Footing the Bill*, London: Royal Institute of Chartered Surveyors.

Bartley, M. (1994) 'Unemployment and ill health: understanding the relationship', *Journal of Epidemiology and Community Health* 48(4): 333–7.

Baxter, C. (1994) 'Sex education in the multi-racial society', in A. Craft (ed.) *Practice Issues in Sexuality and Learning Difficulties*, London: Routledge.

Bayliss, K. (forthcoming) 'Social work values, anti-discriminatory practice and working with older lesbian service users', *Social Work Education*.

Bebbington, A. and Miles, J. (1989) 'The background of children who enter local authority care', *British Journal of Social Work* 19(5): 349–68.

Beck, P., Lazarus, J., Scorer, R., Smith, P. and Routledge, P. (1994) 'Increasing rate of deliberate self-poisoning', *British Medical Journal* 308: 789.

Becker, S. (1997) *Responding to Poverty: The Politics of Cash and Care*, Harlow: Addison Wesley Longman.

Bedics, B. (1994) 'Non-use of prenatal care: implications for social work involvement', *Health and Social Work* 19(2): 84–92.

Bell, E.M. (1961) *The Story of the Hospital Almoner*, London: Faber and Faber.

Bendelow, G. (ed.) (1998) *Emotions in Social Life: Critical Themes and Contemporary Issues*, London: Routledge.

Beresford, B., Sloper, P., Baldwin, S. and Newman, T. (1996) *What Works in Services for Families with a Disabled Child?* Ilford: Barnardos.

Beresford, P. and Croft, S. (1995) 'Time for a new approach to anti-poverty campaigning?', *Poverty* 90, Spring 95: 12–14.

Black, D. and Bowman, C. (1997) 'Community institutional care for frail elderly people', *British Medical Journal* 315: 441–2.

Blackburn, C. (1992) *Improving Health and Welfare Work with Families in Poverty: A Handbook*, Buckingham: Open University Press.

—— (1996) 'Building a poverty perspective into health visiting practice', in P. Bywaters and E. McLeod (eds) *Working for Equality in Health*, London: Routledge.

Blackman, T. and Atkinson, A. (1997) 'Needs targeting and resource allocation in community care', *Policy Studies* 18(2): 125–38.

Blane, D., Brunner, E. and Wilkinson, R. (eds) (1996) *Health and Social Organisation*, London: Routledge.

Blaxter, M. (1990) *Health and Lifestyles*, London: Routledge.

British Medical Association (BMA) (1997) Options for Funding Health Care, London: BMA Health Policy and Economic Research Unit.

BMA and the Law Society (1995) *Assessment of Mental Capacity Guidance for Doctors and Lawyers*, London: BMA, The Law Society.

BMA Health Policy and Economic Research Unit (1998) *Quarterly Bulletin* 13(3), September.

Bond, M. (1999) 'Placing poverty on the agenda of a primary health care team: an evaluation of an action research project', *Health and Social Care in the Community* 7(1): 9–16.

Boneham, M., Williams, K.E., Copeland, J.R.M., McKibbin, P., Wilson, K., Scott, A. and Saunders, P.A. (1997) 'Elderly people from ethnic minorities in Liverpool: mental illness, unmet need and barriers to service use', *Health and Social Care in the Community* 5(3): 173–80.

Boulton, I. (1993) 'Youth homelessness and health care', in K. Fisher and J. Collins (eds) *Homelessness, Health Care and Welfare Provision*, London: Routledge.

Bourgeois, C.G. (1998) 'The impact of AIDS on the life cycle of young gay men', unpublished MA thesis, School of Social Work, McGill University, Montreal, Canada.

Bowling, A. and Windsor, J. (1997) 'Discriminative power of the Health Status Questionnaire 12 in relation to age, sex, and long-standing illness: findings from a survey of households in Great Britain', *Journal of Epidemiology and Community Health* 51: 564–73.

Brannen, J., Dodd, K., Oakley, A. and Storey, P. (1994) *Young People, Health and Family Life*, Buckingham. Open University Press.

British Road Federation (1998) *Item Details*, London: press release ID: 20/98.

Broad, B. (1998) *Young People Leaving Care: Life after the Children Act 1989*, London: Jessica Kingsley.

Bunton, R., Nettleton, S. and Burrows, R. (eds) (1995) *The Sociology of Health Promotion*, London: Routledge.

Burch, R. (1997) 'Alive and Kicking', *Nursing Times* 93(9): 6–12.

Burnard, P. (1995) 'Implications of client-centred counselling for nursing practice', *Nursing Times*, 91(26): 35–7.

Burrows, R., Nettleton, S. and Bunton, R. (1995) 'Sociology and health promotion' in R. Bunton, S. Nettleton and R. Burrows (eds) *The Sociology of Health Promotion*, London: Routledge.

Butler, P. (1998) 'In a sad state', *Guardian* Society 12 August: 23–24.

Butt, J. and Mirza, K. (1996) *Social Care and Black Communities*, London: HMSO.

Bytheway, B. and Furth, A. (1996) 'Asthma', in B. Davey and C. Seale (eds) *Experiencing and Explaining Disease*, Buckingham: Open University Press.

Bywaters, P. (1986) 'Social work and the medical profession: arguments against unconditional collaboration', *British Journal of Social Work* 16: 661–77.

—— (1989) 'Social work and nursing: sisters or rivals?', in R. Taylor and J. Ford (eds) *Social Work and Health Care*, London: Jessica Kingsley.

—— (1991) 'Case-funding and screening for social work in acute general hospitals', *British Journal of Social Work* 21: 19–39.

—— (1996) 'Government, social services departments and the health of children and young people: which way forward?', *British Journal of Social Work* 26: 777–94.

Bywaters, P. and Harris, A. (1998) 'Supporting carers: is practice still sexist?' *Health and Social Care in the Community* 6(6): 458–63.

Bywaters, P. and McLeod, E. (1996a) 'Introduction' in P. Bywaters and E. McLeod (eds) *Working for Equality in Health*, London: Routledge.

—— (1996b) 'Can social work deliver on health?' in P. Bywaters and E. McLeod (eds) *Working for Equality in Health*, London: Routledge.

Calnan, M. and Williams, S. (eds) (1996) *Modern Medicine: Lay Perspectives and Experience*, London: UCL Press.

Cannon, A.G., Semwogerere, A., Lamont, D.W., Hole, O.J., Mallon, E.A., George, W.D. and Gillis, C.R. (1994) 'Relation between socio-economic deprivation and pathological prognostic factors in women with breast cancer', *British Medical Journal* 307: 1054–7.

Carlen, P. (1994) 'The governance of homelessness: legality, lore and lexicon in the agency maintenance of youth homelessness', *Critical Social Policy* 14(2): 18–35.

Carne, C. (1998) 'Sexually transmitted infections', *British Medical Journal* 317: 129–39.

Carr-Hill, R.A., Rice, N. and Roland, M. (1996) 'Socio-economic determinants of rates of consultation in general practice based on the fourth national morbidity survey of general practices', *British Medical Journal* 312: 1008–13.

Carricaburu, D. and Pierret, J. (1995) 'From biographical disruption to biographical reinforcement: the case of HIV-positive men', *Sociology of Health and Illness* 17: 65–88.

Carter, Y.H. and Jones, P.W. (1993) 'Accidents among children under five years old: a general practice-based study in north Staffordshire', *British Journal of General Practice* 43: 159–63.

Cartwright, A. (1991) 'The role of residential and nursing homes in the last year of people's lives', *British Journal of Social Work* 21: 627–45.

Castel, R. (1991) 'From dangerousness to risk', in G. Burchell, C. Gordon and P. Miller (eds) *The Foucault Effect: Studies in Governmentality*, London: Harvester.

Centrepoint (1997) *The Point 1995–96*, London: Centrepoint.

Chadwick, R. and Russell, J., (1989) 'Hospital discharge of frail elderly people: social and ethical considerations in the discharge decision-making process', *Ageing and Society* 9: 277–95.

Challis, L. and Henwood, M. (1994) 'Equity in Community Care', *British Medical Journal* 308: 1496–9.

Charles, N. and Walters, V. (1998) 'Age and gender in women's accounts of their health: interviews with women in south Wales', *Sociology of Health and Illness* 20(3): 331–50.

Claridge, B. and Rivers, P. (1997) *Evaluation of Social Workers Attached to GP Practices*, Derby: University of Derby and Southern Derbyshire Health.

Clark, B. and Davis, A. (1997) 'When money's too tight to mention', *Professional Social Work* March: 12–13.

Clark, D. (ed.) (1993) *The Future for Palliative Care*, Buckingham: Open University Press.

—— (1998) 'The future of palliative care', paper presented at the Palliative Care Conference, Wigan and Leigh Hospice: Wigan.

Clark, D. and Seymour, J. (1998) *Reflections on Palliative Care*, Buckingham: Open University Press.

Clark, D., Hockley, J. and Ahmedzai, S. (eds) (1997) *New Themes in Palliative Care*, Buckingham: Open University Press.

Clark, H., Dyer, S. and Hartman, L. (1996) *Going Home: Older People Leaving Hospital*, Bristol: University of Bristol, The Policy Press.

Clarke, M. (1993) 'Speaking up', *Nursing Times* 89(2), 13 January: 42–4.

Clement-Jones, V. (1985) 'Cancer and beyond: the formation of BACUP', *British Medical Journal* 291: 1021–3.

Cochrane, G.M., Jackson, W.F. and Rees, P. J. (1994) *Asthma – Current Perspectives*, London: Mosby-Wolfe.

Cohen, R. and Wiffen, J. (1996) *Family Support and Anti-Poverty Strategy*, London: Local Government Anti-Poverty Unit.

Conaty, P. and Mayo, E. (1997) *A Commitment to People and Place*, London: New Economics Foundation.

Connor, A. and Tibbitt, J.E. (1988) *Social Workers and Health Care in Hospitals*, Edinburgh: HMSO.

Conrad, P. (1985) 'The meaning of medication: another look at compliance', *Social Science and Medicine* 20(1): 29–37.

Cooper, H. Arber, S. and Smaje, C. (1998a) 'Social class or deprivation? Structural factors and children's limiting long-standing illness in the 1990s', *Sociology of Health and Illness* 20(3): 289–311.

—— (1998b) 'Use of health services by children and young people according to ethnicity and social class: secondary analysis of a national survey', *British Medical Journal* 317: 1047–51.

Coote, A. and Hunter, D.J. (1996) *New Agenda for Health*, London: Institute for Public Policy Research.

Corlyon, J. and McGuire, C. (1997) *Young Parents in Public Care*, London: National Children's Bureau.

Corney, R. (1985) 'The health of clients referred to social workers in an intake team', *Social Science and Medicine* 21(8): 873–8.

Cornwell, J. (1984) *Hard Earned Lives*, London: Tavistock.

Cosis Brown, H. (1998) *Social Work and Sexuality*, Basingstoke: Macmillan.

Cowley, S. (1990) 'Who qualifies for terminal care ?' *Nursing Times* 86(22): 29–31.

Craig, G. (1992) 'Anti-poverty action and research in the UK', *Social Policy and Administration* 26(2): 129–43.

Crawford, R. (1980) 'Healthism and the medicalization of everyday life', *International Journal of Health Services* 10(3): 365–88.

Croft, S. (1996) '"How can I leave them?" Towards an empowering social work practice with women who are dying', in B. Fawcett, M. Galloway and J. Perrins (eds) *Feminism and Social Work in the Year 2000: Conflicts and Controversies*, Bradford: University of Bradford.

—— (1998) 'User involvement in palliative care social work', summary of presentation, Association of Hospice and Specialist Palliative Care Social Workers Annual Conference, St Catherine's College, Cambridge.

Crow, L. (1996) 'Including all of our lives: renewing the social model of disability', in C. Barnes and G. Mercer (1996) *Exploring the Divide: Illness and Disability*, Leeds: The Disability Press.

Cumella, S. (1994) *Care Management in a Primary Healthcare Team*, Birmingham: University of Birmingham Centre for Research and Information into Mental Disability.

Cumella, S., Grattan, E. and Vostanis, P. (1998) 'The mental health of children in homeless families and their contact with health, education and social services', *Health and Social Care in the Community* 6(5): 331–42.

Cumella, S., Le Mesurier, N. and Tomlin, H. (undated) *Social Work in Practice: An evaluation of the care management received by elderly people from social workers based in GP practices in South Worcestershire*, Worcester: The Martley Press.

Curtis, S. and Rees Jones, I. (1998) 'Is there a place for geography in the analysis of health inequality?' *Sociology of Health and Illness* 20(5): 645–72.

Dahlgren, G. and Whitehead, M. (1991) *Policies and Strategies to Promote Social Equity in Health*, Stockholm: Institute for Future Studies.

Davey Smith, G. (1994) 'Increasing inequalities in the health of the nation: government action at last?' *British Medical Journal* 309: 1453–4.

—— (1996) 'Income inequality and mortality: why are they related?' *British Medical Journal* 312: 987–8.

Davey Smith, G., Bartley, M. and Blane, D. (1990) 'The Black Report on socio-economic inequalities in health 10 years on', *British Medical Journal* 301: 373–7.

Davey Smith, G., Morris, J.N. and Shaw, M. (1998a) 'The independent inquiry into inequalities in health', *British Medical Journal* 317: 1465–6.

Davey Smith, G., Hart, C., Hole, D., MacKinnon, P., Gillis, C., Watt, G., Blane, D. and Hawthorne, V. (1998b) 'Education and occupational social class: which is the more important indicator of mortality risk? *Journal of Epidemiology and Community Health* 52: 153–60.

Davey Smith, G., Hart, C., Blane, D. and Hole, D. (1998c) 'Adverse socio-economic conditions in childhood can cause specific adult mortality: prospective observational study', *British Medical Journal* 316: 1631–5.

Davey, B. and Seale, C. (eds) (1996) *Experiencing and Explaining Disease*, Buckingham: Open University.

Davies, D. and Neal, C. (eds) (1996) *Pink Therapy*, Buckingham: Open University.

Davies, M. (ed.) (1997) *The Blackwell Companion to Social Work*, Oxford: Blackwell.

Davies, M. and Connolly, J. (1995a) 'The social worker's role in the hospital, seen through the eyes of other healthcare professionals', *Health and Social Care in the Community* 3(5): 301–9.

—— (1995b) 'Hospital social work and discharge planning: an exploratory study in East Anglia', *Health and Social Care in the Community* 3(6): 363–71.

Davis, A. and Wainwright, S. (1996) 'Poverty work and the mental health services', *Breakthrough* 1(1): 47–56.

Davis, C. L. and Sheldon, F. (1997) 'Therapeutic innovations', in D. Clark, L. Hockley and S. Ahmedzai (eds) *New Themes in Palliative Care*, Buckingham, Open University Press.

Davison, C., Frankel, S. and Davey Smith, G. (1992) 'The limits of lifestyle: reassessing "fatalism" in the popular culture of illness prevention', *Social Science and Medicine* 34(6): 675–85.

Department of Health (DoH) (1989) *Caring for People*, London: DoH.

—— (1991a) *Children Act 1989, Guidance and Regulations, Volume 4: Residential Care*, London: DoH.

—— (1991b) *Patterns and Outcomes in Child Placement*, London: DoH.

—— (1991c) *Children in the Public Care*, London: DoH.

—— (1992) *Health of the Nation*, London: DoH.

—— (1995a) *Variations in Health: What Can the Department of Health and the NHS Do?* London: DoH

—— (1995b) *Nutrition Guidelines for Hospital Catering*, London: DoH.

—— (1997a) *The New NHS: Modern and Dependable*, London: DoH.

—— (1997b) '£30 million for new partnerships in health action zones announced', London: DoH press notice 97/312.

—— (1997c) *Healthy Living Centres*, letter to chief executives, London: DoH.

—— (1998a) 'Our Healthier Nation', London: DoH.

—— (1998b) *Modernising Health and Social Services: National Priorities Guidance 1999/00 – 2001/02*, London: DoH.

—— (1998c) 'Modernising Social Services', London: DoH.

—— (1998d) *Quality Protects: Transforming Children's Services*, London: DoH.

—— (1998e) 'Healthy living centres', report of a seminar held on 2 April 1998, London: DoH.

—— (1998f) *Partnership in Action: New Opportunities for Joint Working between Health and Social Services*, London: DoH.

Department of Health and Social Security (DHSS) (1980) 'Inequalities in health', report of a research working group, London: DHSS.

Department of Social Security (DSS) (1997a) *DS2A Special Rules October 1997*, London: DSS.

—— (1997b) *DLAIA Audit October 1997*, notes, London: DSS.

Department of the Environment, Transport and the Regions (DETR) (1998a) *Modern Local Government – In Touch with the People*, London: DETR.

—— (1998b) 'EU ministers slash lorry and bus emissions by 60%', London: DETR press release 1114, 21 December.

—— (1998c) 'Europe breathes more easily', London: DETR press release 490/ENV, 16 June.

—— (1999) 'Particles in the air – an international problem', London: DETR press release 27, 13 January.

Dhooper, S. (1990) 'Family coping with the crisis of a heart attack', in K. Davidson and S. Clarke (eds) *Social Work in Health Care: A Handbook for Practice*, New York: Haworth Press.

Dinsdale, P. (1998) 'Pilot lights new way forward', *Guardian* 4 February: 7.

Dobash, R.E. and Dobash, R.P. (1980) *Violence against Wives*, Shepton Mallet, Somerset: Open Books.

—— (1992) *Women, Violence and Social Change*, London: Routledge.

Dockery, D., Arden Pope, C., Xu, X., Spengler, J., Ware, J., Fay, M., Ferris, B. and Speizer, F. (1993) 'An association between air pollution and mortality in six US cities', *New England Journal of Medicine* 329(24): 1753–60.

Douglas, J. (1996) 'Developing with Black and ethnic minority communities, health promotion strategies which address social inequalities', in P. Bywaters and E. McLeod (eds) *Working for Equality in Health*, London: Routledge.

Doyal, L. (1995) *What Makes Women Sick?* Basingstoke: Macmillan.

Drakeford, M. (1997) 'The poverty of privatisation: poorest customers of the privatised gas, water and electricity industries', *Critical Social Policy* 17(2): 115–32.

—— (1998) 'Poverty and community care', in A. Symonds and A. Kelly (eds) *The Social Construction of Community Care*, Basingstoke: Macmillan.

Drakeford, M. and Hudson, B. (1994) *Credit Unions and Barnardos: A Partnership to Tackle Poverty*, Cardiff: Barnardos.

Drever, F. and Whitehead, M. (eds) (1997) *Health Inequalities*, London: HMSO.

Dunn, M. and McClusky, J. (1997) *NCH Action for Children 98 Factfile*, London: NCH Action for Children.

Dunning, A. (1995) *Citizen Advocacy with Older People*, London: Centre for Policy on Ageing.

Editorial (1995) 'Changing Patterns of conssultation in general practices: fouth national morbidity study, 1991–1992', *British Journal of General Practice* June: 283–5.

Edwards, P. and Kenny, D. (1997) *Community Care Trends (1997) Report: The Impact of Funding on Local Authorities*, London: Local Government Management Board.

Eiser, C., Zoritch, B., Hiller, J., Havermans, T. and Billig, S. (1995) 'Routine stresses in caring for a child with cystic fibrosis', *Journal of Psychosomatic Research* 39(5): 641–6.

Erskine, A. (1996) 'The burden of risk: who dies because of cars?' *Social Policy and Administration* 30(2): 43–57.

Evans, C. (1996) 'Service users acting as agents of change', in P. Bywaters and E. McLeod (eds) *Working for Equality in Health*, London: Routledge.

Evans, C. and Fisher, M. (1999) 'Collaborative evaluations with service users: moving towards user-controlled research' in I. Shaw and J. Lishman (eds) *Evaluation and Social Work Practice*, London: Sage.

Expert Advisory Group on Cancer (1995) *A Policy Framework for Commissioning Cancer Services*, report to the chief medical officers of England and Wales, London: Department of Health.

Fentiman, I.S., Tirelli, U., Monfardini, S., Schneider, M., Festen, J., Cognetti, F. and Aapro, M.S. (1990) 'Cancer in the elderly, why so badly treated?', *The Lancet* 335: 1020–2.

Fenton, S. (1997) *Ethnicity and Mental Health*, Bristol: University of Bristol, School for Policy Studies.

Ferrie, J.E., Shipley, M.J., Marmot, M.G., Stansfield, S. and Davey Smith, G. (1995) 'Health effects of anticipation of job change and non-employment: longitudinal data from the Whitehall II study', *British Medical Journal* 311: 1264–9.

Field, D. and James, N. (1993) 'Where and how people die', in D. Clark (ed.) *The Future for Palliative Care*, Buckingham: Open University Press.

Field, D., Hockey, J. and Small, N. (eds) (1997) *Death, Gender and Ethnicity*, London: Routledge.

Fimister, G. (1994) *Anti-Poverty Strategy: Origins and Options*, London: Local Government Anti-Poverty Unit.

Firth, P. (1998) 'Whose hospice is it anyway? A perspective from a social worker', paper presented at the Help the Hospices annual national conference, London.

Fisher, K. and Collins, J. (eds) (1993) *Homelessness, Healthcare and Welfare Provision*, London: Routledge.

Foster, P. (1995) *Women and the Health Care Industry: An Unhealthy Relationship*, Buckingham: Open University Press.

French, J. (1995) 'Charging elders: perverse incentives and poverty', *Critical Social Policy* 44/45: 96–106.

Friends of the Earth (FOE) (1995) *Prescription for Change: Health and the Environment*, London: FOE.

—— (1998) 'FOE dismisses road lobby's desperate attack on new law to reduce traffic', London: FOE press release 15 January 98.

Fruin, D. (1998) *A Matter of Chance for Carers*, London: Department of Health.

Gabe, J., Kelleher, D. and Williams, G. (1994) *Challenging Medicine*, London: Routledge.

Gannon, L. (1998) 'The impact of medical and sexual politics on women's health', *Feminism and Psychology* 8(3): 285–302.

Gardner, K., Regan, M., Mahoney, G. and Thompson, A. (1996) *Asthma Nitrogen Dioxide Community Monitoring Project*, Liverpool: Friends of the Earth.

Garnett L. (1992) *Leaving Care and After*, London: NCB.

Gaze, H. (1998) 'Learning disabled but breast aware', *Healthlines* May: 24–5.

Gibbs, G. (1995) 'Nurses in private nursing homes: a study of their knowledge and attitudes to pain management in palliative care', *Palliative Medicine* 9: 245–53.

Gibbs, L.M.E., Addington-Hall, J. and Gibbs, J.S.R. (1998) 'Dying from heart failure: lessons from palliative care', *British Medical Journal* 317: 961–2.

Gillam, S. (1992) 'Provision of health promotion clinics in relation to population need: another example of the inverse care law?' *British Journal of General Practice* 42: 54–6.

Ginn, J. (1993) 'Grey power: age-based organisations' response to structured inequalities', *Critical Social Policy* 38: 23–47.

Glassner, B. (1995) 'In the name of health', in R. Bunton, S. Nettleton and R. Burrows (eds) *The Sociology of Health Promotion*, London: Routledge.

Glennerster, H. and Midgeley, J. (eds) (1991) *The Radical Right and the Welfare State: An International Reassessment*, London: Harvester Wheatsheaf/Barnes and Noble Books.

Glickman, M. (1996) *Palliative Care in the Hospital Setting*, London: National Council for Hospice and Specialist Palliative Care Services.

Godfrey, M. and Moore, J. (1996) *Hospital Discharge: User, Carer and Professional Perspectives*, Leeds: Nuffield Institute for Health, University of Leeds.

Goldstein, R. and Rivers, P. (1996) 'The medication role of informal carers', *Health and Social Care in the Community* 4(3): 150–8.

Gottlieb, S. (1998) 'AIDS deaths fall by nearly one half', *British Medical Journal* 317: 4.

Grace, V.M. (1991) 'The marketing of empowerment and the construction of the health consumer: a critique of health promotion', *International Journal of Health Services* 21(2): 329–43.

Graham, H. (1984) *Women, Health and the Family*, Brighton: Wheatsheaf.

—— (1987) 'Women's smoking and family health', *Social Science and Medicine* 25(1): 474–86.

—— (1993) *Health and Hardship in Women's Lives*, London: Harvester Wheatsheaf.

—— (1995) 'Diversity, inequality and official data: some problems of method and measurement in Britain', *Health and Social Care in the Community* 3: 9–18.

—— (1996) 'Researching women's health work: a study of the lifestyles of mothers on income support', in P. Bywaters and E. McLeod (eds) *Working for Equality in Health*, London: Routledge.

Graham, H.J. and Firth, J. (1992) 'Home accidents in older people: the role of the primary health care team', *British Medical Journal* 305: 30–2.

Grande, G.E., Addington-Hall, J.M. and Todd, C.J. (1998) 'Place of death and access to home care services: are certain patient groups at a disadvantage?' *Social Science and Medicine* 47(5): 565–79.

Grattan, E., Le Mesurier, N. and Cumella, S. (1995) *Practitioner Alliances in Primary Care*, Birmingham: University of Birmingham Centre for Research and Information into Mental Disability.

Gray, A. (ed.) (1993) *World Health and Disease*, Buckingham: Open University Press.

Green, J. (1995) 'Accidents and the risk society: some problems with prevention', in R. Bunton, S. Nettleton and R. Burrows (eds) *The Sociology of Health Promotion*, London: Routledge.

Green, R. (1997) *Community Action against Poverty*, Hackney, London: The Kingsmead Kabin, 9, Kingsmead Way, Kingsmead Estate, E9 5QG.

Greenhalgh, T., Helman, C. and Mu'min Chowdhury, A. (1998) 'Health beliefs and folk models of diabetes in British Bangladeshis: a qualitative study', *British Medical Journal* 316: 978–83.

Gunaratnam, Y. (1997) 'Culture is not enough: a critique of multiculturalism in palliative care', in D. Field, J. Hockey and N. Small (eds) *Death, Gender and Ethnicity*, London: Routledge.

—— (1998) 'Rethinking multi-cultural service provision', *Hospice Bulletin*, 6(2): 7–8.

Gunnell, D.J., Peters, T.J., Kammerling, R.M. and Brooks, J. (1995) 'Relation between parasuicide, suicide, psychiatric admissions and socio-economic deprivation', *British Medical Journal* 311: 226–30.

Hague, G. and Malos, E. (1994) *Domestic Violence: Action for Change*, Cheltenham: New Clarion Press.

Hall, A., Fallowfield, L.J. and A'Hern, R.P. (1996) 'When breast cancer recurs: a 3-year prospective study of psychological morbidity', *The Breast Journal* 2(3): 197–203.

Hann, A. (1995) 'Screening women for cancer: a time for reappraisal?' *Critical Social Policy* 44/45: 183–92.

Hannay, D.R. (1980) 'The illness iceberg and trivial consultations', *Journal of the Royal College of General Practitioners* 30: 551–4.

Hansard (1997) *Written Answers*, 10 March, cols 99–100: 99, London: HMSO.

Harding, T. (1997) *A Life Worth Living*, London: Help the Aged.

Harding, T., Meredith, B. and Wistow, G. (1996) 'Looking to the future', in T. Harding, B. Meredith and G. Wistow (eds) *Options for Long-term Care: Economic, Social and Ethical Choices*, London: HMSO.

Harris, L. (1990) 'The disadvantaged dying', *Nursing Times* 86(22): 26–29.

Harvey, A. and Robertson, G. (1995) *Survey of Charges for Social Care 1993–5*, London: Local Government Anti-Poverty Unit.

Haworth, M., Lennard, R., Sadiq, A. and Smith, M. (1997) 'Asian interpreters and palliative care', *Palliative Medicine Research Abstracts*, 11: 77.

Health Advisory Service (HAS) 2000 (1998) *Not Because They are Old: An independent inquiry into the care of older people on acute wards in general hospitals*, London: HAS 2000.

Health Policy Network (1995) *In Practice: The NHS Market*, Banbury: NHS Consultants Association in conjunction with NHS Support Federation.

—— (1996) *Health Care: Private Corporations or Public Service? The Americanisation of the NHS*, Banbury: NHS Consultants Association in conjunction with NHS Support Federation and the Public Health Alliance.

Hearn, J. and Higginson, I.J. (1998) 'Do specialist palliative care teams improve outcomes for cancer patients? A systematic literature review', *Palliative Medicine* 12: 317–22.

Heaven, C.M. and Maguire, P. (1997) 'Disclosure of concerns by hospice patients and their identification by nurses', *Palliative Medicine* 11: 283–90.

Henwood, M. (1991) 'No sense of urgency: age discrimination in health care', *Critical Public Health* 2: 4–14.

—— (1995) 'Tipping the balance: the implications of changes in acute health care for patients and their families', *Research Paper 19*, Birmingham: National Association of Health Authorities and Trusts.

—— (1997) 'Discharging responsibilities', *Community Care* Inside, 25 September–1 October: 7.

Henwood, M., Hardy, B., Hudson, B. and Wistow, G. (1997) *Inter-agency Collaboration: Hospital Discharge and Continuing Care Sub-study*, Leeds: University of Leeds, Nuffield Institute for Health, Community Care Division.

Hepworth, M. (1995) 'Positive ageing: what is the message?', in R. Bunton, S. Nettleton and R. Burrows (eds) *The Sociology of Health Promotion*, London: Routledge.

Herbert, A. and Kempson, E. (1996) *Credit Use among Ethnic Minorities*, London: Policy Studies Institute.

Higginson, I. (1993) 'Quality, costs and contracts of care', in D. Clark (ed.) *The Future for Palliative Care*, Buckingham: Open University Press.

Higginson, I., Webb, D. and Lessof, L. (1994) 'Reducing hospital beds for patients with advanced cancer', *The Lancet* 344: 409.

HM Treasury (1998a) 'Taskforce to look at how banks can help credit unions', news release 123/98, 28 July, London: HM Treasury.

—— (1998b) 'Banks/credit unions Taskforce: membership announced', news release 155/98, 22 September, London: HM Treasury.

Hockley, J. (1997) 'The evolution of the hospice approach', in D. Clark, J. Hockley and S. Ahmedzai (eds) *New Themes in Palliative Care*, Buckingham: Open University Press.

Hoff, M.D. (1997) 'The physical environment: expanding social work knowledge and practice skills to the movement for a sustainable future', paper presented at a conference on Culture and Identity: Social Work in a Changing Europe, Dublin: International Federation of Social Workers (Europe) and European Association of Schools of Social Work.

Holtermann, S. (1995) *All Our Futures*, Ilford: Barnardos.

House of Commons Health Committee (1996) *Long-term Care: Future Provision and Funding*, third report, session 1995–1996, HC 59–1, London: HMSO.

Howells, G. (1986) 'Are the medical needs of mentally handicapped adults being met?' *Journal of the Royal College of General Practitioners* 36: 449–53.

Howes, K. (1997) *Deaths of People Alone*, London: Centre for Policy on Ageing, Help the Aged.

Hudson, B., Newman, T. and Drakeford, M. (1994) 'Developing a credit union – a community-based response to poverty', *Critical Social Policy* 14: 117–24.

Hughes, G. and Lewis, G. (eds) (1998) *Unsettling Welfare: The Reconstruction of Social Policy*, London: Routledge in association with the Open University.

Hume, M., Moore. H. And Woodcock, S. (1998) 'Government Recognition', *Perspectives* 69: 3.

Hutton, W. (1998) 'The state we should be in', *Marxism Today* Special Issue, November/December: 34–7.

Imtiaz, S. and Johnson, M.R.D. (1993) *Health Care Provision and the Kashmiri Population of Peterborough: An Initial Investigation of Issues of Concern*, Coventry: University of Warwick, Centre for Research in Ethnic Relations.

Income Data Services (1998) *Public Sector Labour Market Survey*, London: Income Data Services.

Independent Inquiry (1998) *Independent Inquiry into Inequalities in Health*, London: Stationery Office.

Inman, P. (1999) 'No place like home', *Guardian* January 16, Jobs and Money: 2–3.

Jackson, A. and Eve, A. (eds) (1998) *1998 Directory of Hospice and Palliative Care Services*, London: The Hospice Information Service at St Christopher's.

Jacobs, M. (1998) *The Third Way*, The Fabian Society.

Johnson, P. (1997) *Inequality in the UK*, London: Institute of Fiscal Studies.

Johnson, M. and Sangster, D. (1996) *Health Needs of African Caribbean People in Peterborough*, Peterborough: North West Anglia Health.

Johnson, S. and Rogaly, B. (1997) *Microfinance and Poverty Reduction*, Oxford: Oxfam and London: Actionaid.

Jones, A. (1997) 'Death, poetry, psychotherapy and clinical supervision (the contribution of psychodynamic psychotherapy to palliative care nursing)', *Journal of Advanced Nursing* 25(2): 238–44.

Jones, C. (1997) 'Poverty', in M. Davies (ed.) *Blackwell Companion to Social Work*, Oxford: Blackwell.

Jones, L. (1994) *The Social Context of Health and Health Work*, Basingstoke: Macmillan.

Jones, L. and Sidell, M. (eds) (1997) *The Challenge of Promoting Health: Exploration and Action*, Basingstoke: Macmillan.

Jones, P.A. (1999) *Towards Sustainable Credit Union Development*, Manchester: Association of British Credit Unions Ltd.

Joseph Rowntree Foundation (1995a) 'Unleashing the potential: bringing residents to the centre of regeneration', York: Joseph Rowntree Foundation, *Policy Options*, supplement to *Housing Research Summary* No. 12.

—— (1995b) *Inquiry into Income and Wealth*, York: Joseph Rowntree Foundation.

—— (1997) 'Living well into old age', *Findings*, Social Care Research 95, York: Joseph Rowntree Foundation.

—— (1998a) 'The cost of childhood disability', *Findings*, July, York: Joseph Rowntree Foundation.

—— (1998b) 'The number and characteristics of families with more than one disabled child', *Findings*, February, York: Joseph Rowntree Foundation.

—— (1998c) 'The importance of "low level" preventative services to older people', *Findings*, July, York: Joseph Rowntree Foundation.

Judge, K. and Benzeval, M. (1993) 'Health inequalities: new concerns about children of single mothers', *British Medical Journal* 306: 677–80.

Kai, J. (1996) 'Parents' difficulties and information needs in coping with acute illness in pre-school children: a qualitative study', *British Medical Journal* 313: 987–90.

Kaplan, S.H., Greenfield, S. and Ware, J.E. (1989) 'Assessing the effects of physician-patient interactions on the outcomes of chronic disease', *Medical Care* 27 (supplement 3): 110–27.

Kastenbaum, R. (1993) 'Dame Cicely Saunders: An Omega Interview', *OMEGA* 27(4): 263–9.

Katsouyanni, L., Touloumi, G., Spix, C., Schwartz, J., Balducci, F., Medina, S., Rossi, G., Wojtyniak, B., Sunyer, J., Bacharova, L., Schouten, J.P., Ponka, A. and Anderson, H.R. (1997) 'Short-term effects of ambient sulphur dioxide and particulate matter on mortality in 12 European cities: results from time series data from the APEA project', *British Medical Journal* 314: 1658–63.

Kelly, M.P. and Field, D. (1996) 'Medical sociology, chronic illness and the body', *Sociology of Health and Illness* 18(2): 241–57.

Kempson, E. (1994) 'Outside the banking system: a review of households without a current account', *Social Security Advisory Committee Research Paper 6*, London: HMSO.

—— (1996) *Life on a Low Income*, York: Joseph Rowntree Foundation.

Kendrick, K. (1995a) 'Codes of professional conduct and the dilemmas of professional practice', in K. Soothill, L. Mackay and C. Webb (eds) *Interprofessional Relations in Health Care*, London: Edward Arnold.

—— (1995b) 'Nurses and doctors: a problem of partnership', in K. Soothill, L. Mackay and C. Webb *Interprofessional Relations in Health Care*, London: Edward Arnold.

Khan, S. (1997) *Today's Concerns and Bleak Tomorrows*, London: Service Access to Minority Ethnic Communities.

Killeen, J. (1996) *Advocacy and Dementia*, Edinburgh: Alzheimer's Scotland Action on Dementia.

King, E. (1993) *Safety in Numbers*, London: Cassell.

Komaromy, C. (1998) 'The sight and sound of death', paper presented at the 4th International Conference on the Social Context of Death, Dying and Disposal, Glasgow: Caledonian University.

Labonte, R. (1997) 'Econology: integrating health and sustainable development. Guiding principles for decision-making', in M. Sidell, L. Jones, J. Katz and A. Peberdy (eds) *Debates and Dilemmas in Promoting Health: A Reader*, Basingstoke: Macmillan.

Labour Party (1995) *Peace at Home: A Labour Party Consultation on the Elimination of Domestic Violence and Sexual Violence against Women*, London: Labour Party.

Langan, M. (1998) *Welfare: Needs, Rights and Risks*, London: Routledge in association with the Open University.

Laungani, P. (1992) *It Shouldn't Happen To A Patient*, London: Whitting and Birch.

Lawton, J. (1998) 'Contemporary hospice care: the sequestration of the unbounded body and dirty dying', *Sociology of Health and Illness* 20(2): 121–43.

Le Mesurier, N. and Cumella, S. (1996) *Social Work at Tile Hill Primary Care Services*, Coventry: Tile Hill Primary Health Care Services and Coventry SSD.

Lester, D. (1994) 'Evaluating the effectiveness of the Samaritans in England and Wales', *International Journal of Health Sciences* 5(2): 73–4.

Levitas, R. (1996) 'The concept of social exclusion and the new Durkheimian hegemony', *Critical Social Policy* 16(1): 5–20.

Lewis, G. (ed.) (1998) *Forming Nation: Framing Welfare*, London: Routledge in association with the Open University.

Lewis, J. and Glennerster, H. (1996) *Implementing the New Community Care*, Buckingham: Open University Press.

Littlechild, R. (1996) 'Investigating the mental health needs of the South Asian community in the Small Heath constituency of Birmingham', *Social Services Research* 3: 1–11.

Littlewood, J. (1992) *Aspects of Grief*, London: Routledge.

Liverpool Friends of the Earth and Vauxhall Health Forum (1993) *Ambient Nitrogen Dioxide Levels in the Vauxhall Area of Liverpool*, Liverpool: FOE.

Liverpool Health Authority (1997) *Liverpool Public Health Annual Report 1997*, Liverpool: Liverpool Health Authority.

Llewellin, S. and Murdock, A. (1996) *Saving the Day*, London: CHAR.

Local Government Anti-Poverty Unit (1996a) *In Kind ... or in Cash: Section 17 and Support for Children in Poverty*, London: Association of Metropolitan Authorities.

—— (1996b) *Partnerships against Poverty*, London: Local Government Management Board.

London Lighthouse (1998) *Services at Lighthouse*, London: London Lighthouse.

Lymbery, M. (1998) 'Care management and professional autonomy: the impact of community care legislation on social work with older people', *British Journal of Social Work* 28(6): 863–78.

Mackay, L., Soothill, K. and Webb, C. (1995) 'Troubled times: the context for interprofessional collaboration?', in L. Mackay, K. Soothill and C. Webb (eds) *Interprofessional Relations in Health Care*, London: Edward Arnold.

Mackenbach, J.P. and Kunst, A.E. (1997) 'Measuring the magnitude of socio-economic inequalities in health: an overview of available measures illustrated with two examples from Europe', *Social Science and Medicine*, 44(6): 757–71.

Mackenbach, J.P., Bouvier-Cole, M.H. and Jougla, E. (1990) '"Avoidable" mortality and health services: a review of aggregate data studies', *Journal of Epidemiology and Community Health* 44: 106–11.

Mann, J. (1991) 'The new health care paradigm', *Focus: A Guide to AIDS Research and Counselling* 6(3): 1–2.

Mark, I. (1996) 'Ill-staffed by moonlight (implications of trend to ask nurses to work extra shifts to cover shortages)', *Health Service Journal* 23 May: 17.

Marks, L. (1992) 'Discharging patients or responsibilities? Acute hospital discharge and elderly people', in A. Harrison and D. Bruscini (eds) *Health Care UK 1991*, London: Kings Fund Institute.

Marmot, M. and Shipley, M.J. (1996) 'Do socio-economic differences in mortality persist after retirement? 25-year follow-up of civil servants from the first Whitehall study', *British Medical Journal* 313: 1177–80.

Marmot, M., Shipley, M. and Rose, G. (1984) 'Inequalities in death: specific explanations of a general pattern', *The Lancet*, 5 May: 1003–6.

Marxism Today (1998) Special Issue, November/December.

Mason, A. and Palmer, A. (1996) *Queerbashing: A National Survey of Hate Crimes against Lesbians and Gay Men*, London: Stonewall.

Mayall, B. (1993) 'Keeping healthy at home and school: "It's my body, so it's my job"', *Sociology of Health and Illness* 15 (4): 464–87.

Mayo, M. (1997) 'Partnerships for regeneration and community development: some opportunities, challenges and constraints', *Critical Social Policy* 17(3): 3–26.

Mayor, S. (1995) 'Breathing easier ... nurse-led discharge planning could remedy dangerous gaps in the management and follow-up of asthma patients', *Nursing Times* 91, 4–10 October (40): 18.

McCann, M. and Wisener, A. (1989/90) 'Relaxation Skills', Practice 3 and 4: 316–26.

McCarthy, M., Addington-Hall, J. and Ley, M. (1997) 'Communication and choice in dying from heart disease', *Journal of the Royal Society of Medicine* 90: 128–31.

McCartney, A. (1995) *Teleconferencing Support Group: Results of Evaluation*, London: C4 Ward, Breast Cancer Care.

McClusky, J. and Abrahams, C. (1998) *Factfile 99*, London: NCH Action for Children.

McHugh, S. (1996) *Not at My Age: Why the Present Breast Screening System is Failing Women Aged 65 or Over*, London: Age Concern England.

McKee, L. (1993) 'Poor children in rich countries: markets fail children', *British Medical Journal* 307: 1575–6.

McKeown, T. (1979) *The Role of Medicine: Dream, Mirage or Nemesis*, Oxford: Blackwell.

McLees, S. (1996) *Palliative Care for Black and Ethnic Minority Groups*, Aylesbury, Buckinghamshire: Aylesbury Vale Healthcare Trust.

McLeod, E. (1994) *Women's Experience of Feminist Therapy and Counselling*, Buckingham: Open University Press.

—— (1995a) 'The strategic importance of hospital social work', *Social Work and Social Sciences Review* 6(1): 19–31.

—— (1995b) 'Patients in inter-professional practice', in K. Soothill, L. Mackay and C. Webb (eds) *Interprofessional Relations in Health Care*, London: Edward Arnold.

—— (1997) 'Care management: information access and older people', *Practice* 9(1): 33–43.

—— (1998) 'Women with secondary breast cancer: developing self-help support groups', *Practice* 10(3): 13–26.

—— (forthcoming) *Older Women With Advanced Breast Cancer: Their Experience of a Self-help Support Group*, Birmingham: Birmingham Age Concern.

McLeod, E. and Bywaters, P. (1999) 'Tackling inequalities in physical health: a new objective for social work', *British Journal of Social Work* 29(4): 547–66.

McNaught, A. (1987) *Health Action and Ethnic Minorities*, London: Bedford Square Press.

McNeish, D. and Roberts, H. (1995) *Playing it Safe*, Ilford: Barnardos.

Mead, D. (1997) 'Youth homelessness – let's make a difference', *Homelessness Update*, London: NCH Action for Children.

Means, R. (1997) 'Home, independence and community care: time for a wider vision', *Policy and Politics* 25(4): 409–19.

Means, R. and Smith, R. (1994) *Community Care, Policy and Practice*, Basingstoke: Macmillan.

—— (1998) *Community Care, Policy and Practice*, Basingstoke, Macmillan.

Means, R., Brenton, M. Harrison, L. and Heywood, F. (1997) *Making Partnerships Work in Community Care: A Guide for Practitioners in Housing, Health and Social Services*, Bristol: Policy Press.

Midlands Pensioner Convention (1993) *West Midlands Pensioner* No. 42, Autumn.

—— (1996) *West Midlands Pensioner* No. 54, Winter.

Modood, T., Berthoud, R., Lakey, J., Nazroo, J., Virdee, S. and Beishon, S. (1997) *Ethnic Minorities in Britain: Diversity and Disadvantage*, London: Policy Studies Institute.

Mohan, J. (1995) *A National Health Service?*, London: Macmillan.

Mooney, J. (1994) *The Hidden Figure: Domestic Violence in North London*, London: London Borough of Islington, Policy and Crime Prevention Unit.

Moore, R. and Harrison, S. (1995) 'In poor health: socioeconomic status and health chances – a review of the literature', *Social Sciences in Health* 1(4): 221–35.

MORI for Cancer Relief Macmillan Fund (1992) *The Social Impact of Cancer*, London: Cancer Relief Macmillan Fund.

Morley, R. and Mullender, A. (1994) *Preventing Domestic Violence to Women*, Policy Research Group, Crime Prevention Series Paper 48, London: Home Office Policy Department.

Morris, J. (1993) *Independent Lives*, Basingstoke: Macmillan.

Mullender, A. (1996) *Rethinking Domestic Violence: The Social Work and Probation Response*, London: Routledge.

—— (1997) 'Domestic violence and social work: the challenge to change', *Critical Social Policy* 17(1): 53–75.

Mullender, A. and Humphreys, C. (1998) Local Government Association briefing paper: 'Domestic violence and child abuse, policy and practice issues for local authorities and other agencies', London: Local Government Association.

Mullender, A. and Perrott, S. (1998) 'Social work and organisations', in R. Adams, L. Dominelli and M. Payne (eds) *Social Work: Themes, Issues and Critical Debates*, Basingstoke: Macmillan.

Murray, C. (1990) *The Emerging British Underclass*, London: Institute of Economic Affairs.

Naish, J. (1995) 'Recruitment crisis returns (fears about a nursing supply shortage)', *Nursing Management* January, 1(8): 6–7.

National Asthma Campaign (1999) *Asthma Agenda*, http.www.asthma.org.uk/postcard.html

National Council for Hospice and Specialist Palliative Care Services (NCHSPCS) (1995a) *Opening Doors: Improving Access to Hospice and Specialist Palliative Care Services by Members of the Black and Ethnic Minority Communities*, London: NCHSPCS.

—— (1995b) *Information Exchange* No. 14, London: NCHSPCS.

—— (1998) *Promoting Partnership: Planning and Managing Community Palliative Care*, London: NCHSPCS.

Naylor, M. D. (1990) 'Comprehensive discharge planning for hospitalised elderly: a pilot study', *Nursing Research* 39, May–June, (3): 156–61.

Nazroo, J. (1997) *The Health of Britain's Ethnic Minorities*, London: Policy Studies Institute.

Neill, J. and Williams, J. (1992) *Leaving Hospital; Elderly People and their Discharge to Community Care*, London: National Institute of Social Work, Department of Health and Social Security.

Nettleton, S. (1996) 'Women and the new paradigm of health and medicine', *Critical Social Policy* 48: 33–53.

Nettleton, S. and Bunton, R. (1995) 'Sociological critiques of health promotion', in R. Bunton, S. Nettleton and R. Burrows (eds) *The Sociology of Health Promotion*, London: Routledge.

Newtown/South Aston Credit Union Ltd (1997) *Credit Union News*, Birmingham: Newtown/South Aston Credit Union Ltd.

NHS Centre for Reviews and Dissemination (1996) 'Ethnicity and Health', *CRD Report 5*, York: University of York.

NHS Executive (1995) *The Transfer of Frail Older NHS Patients to Other Long-stay Settings*, NSC 19998/048, London: Department of Health.

—— (1996) *Executive Letter*, EL (96) 85.

—— (1998) Health Service Circular *Palliative Care*, HSC 1998/115.

—— (1998) *Planning for Better Health and Better Health Care*, York: NHS Executive HSC 1998/169.

Oakley, A. (1984) *Becoming a Mother*, Oxford: Martin Robertson.

—— (1989) 'Smoking in pregnancy; smokescreen or risk factor? Towards a materialist analysis', *Sociology of Health and Illness* 11(4): 311–35.

Ogden, R.D. and Young, M.G. (1998) 'Euthanasia and assisted suicide: a survey of registered social workers in British Columbia', *British Journal of Social Work* 28(2): 161–77.

Oliver, M. (1990) *The Politics of Disablement*, Basingstoke: Macmillan.

Oliviere, D., Hargreaves, R. and Monroe, B. (1998) *Good Practices in Palliative Care*, Aldershot: Ashgate Arena.

O'Neill, D. (1996) 'Health care for older people: ageism and equality', in P. Bywaters and E. McLeod (eds) *Working for Equality in Health*, London: Routledge.

Ottewill, R., Wall, A. and Yates, J. (1996) 'The "right to be clean": an analysis of the Kirklees home bathing service', *Health and Social Care in the Community* 4(6): 377–80.

Oxenham, D. and Boyd, K. (1998) 'Voluntary euthanasia in terminal illness', in D. Clark, J. Hockley and S. Ahmedzai (eds) *New Themes in Palliative Care*, Buckingham: Open University Press.

Painter, K. (1991) *Wife Rage, Marriage and the Law, Survey Report: Key Findings and Recommendations*, Manchester: Department of Social Policy and Social Work.

Paris, J. and Player, D. (1993) 'Citizens advice in general practice', *British Medical Journal* 306: 1518–20.

Parsons, S. (1997) 'Changing times', *Lighthouse News*, London: London Lighthouse.

Parton, N. (ed.) (1996) *Social Theory, Social Change and Social Work*, London: Routledge.

—— (1997) *Child Protection and Family Support*, London: Routledge.

Payne, D. (1998) 'Panic stations: can the government's new strategy halt the impending catastrophe in nurse recruitment?', *Nursing Times* 94(39): 12–13.

Penhale, B. (1997) 'Towards effective discharge planning', *Health Care in Later Life* 2(1): 46–57.

Perham, L., Winterton, A., Ballard, J., Ewing, M., Lawrence, J. and McCafferty, C. (1998) Early Day Motion No. 606 *Breast Cancer Screening for Women Over 65*, 11 February 1998, London: Randall's Parliamentary Service.

Petticrew, M., McKee, M. and Jones, J. (1993) 'Coronary artery surgery: are women discriminated against?', *British Medical Journal* 306: 1164–6.

Pettinger, N. (1998) 'Age-old myths', *Health Service Journal* 27 August: 24–5.

Phillimore, P. and Moffatt, S. (1994) 'Discounted knowledge: local experience, environmental pollution and health', in J. Popay and G. Williams (eds) *Researching the People's Health*, London: Routledge.

Pinder, R. (1996) 'Sick-but-fit or fit-but-sick? Ambiguity and identity at the workplace', in C. Barnes and G. Mercer *Exploring the Divide: Illness and Disability*, Leeds: The Disability Press.

Pollock, K. (1995) 'Attitude of mind as a means of resisting illness', in A. Radley (ed.) *Worlds of Illness*, London: Routledge.

Popay, J. (1992) 'My health is all right but I'm just tired all the time': women's experience of ill health', in H. Roberts (ed.) *Women's Health Matters*, London: Routledge.

Popay, J., Bartley, M. and Owen, C. (1993) 'Gender inequalities in health, social position, affective disorders and minor physical morbidity', *Social Science and Medicine* 36(1): 21–32.

Positively Women (1994) *Women Like Us*, London: Positively Women.

Pound, P., Gompertz, P. and Ebrahim, S. (1998) 'Illness in the context of older age: the case of stroke', *Sociology of Health and Illness* 20(4): 489–506.

Power, C. and Matthews, S. (1997) 'Origins of health inequalities in a national population sample', *The Lancet* 350: 1584–9.

Power, C., Matthews, S. and Manor, O. (1996) 'Inequalities in self-rated health in the 1958 birth cohort: lifetime social circumstances or social mobility?' *British Medical Journal* 313: 449–53.

—— (1998) 'Inequalities in self-rated health: explanations from different stages of life', *The Lancet* 351: 1009–14.

Quick, A. (1991) *Unequal Risks – Accidents and Social Policy*, London: Socialist Health Association.

Quick, A. and Wilkinson, R. (1991) *Income and Health*, London: Socialist Health Association.

Qureshi, H. and Walker, A. (1989) *The Caring Relationship*, Basingstoke: Macmillan.

Rachman, R. (1993) 'The role of social work in discharge planning', *Health and Social Care*, 1: 105–13.

—— (1995) 'Community care: changing the role of hospital social work', *Health and Social Care in the Community* 3: 163–72.

Raleigh, V.S., Bulusu, L. and Balarajan, R. (1990) 'Suicides among immigrants from the Indian sub-continent', *British Journal of Psychiatry* 156: 46–50.

Raleigh, V.S. and Balarajan, R. (1992) 'Suicide and self-harming among Indians and West Indians in England and Wales', *British Journal of Psychiatry* 161: 365–8.

Ranade, W. (1998) *Markets and Health Care*, London: Longman.

Rathbone, G., Horsley, S. and Goacher, J. (1994) 'A self-evaluated assessment for seriously ill hospice patients', *Palliative Medicine* 8: 29–34.

Reading, R., Colver, A., Openshaw, S. and Jarvis, S. (1994) 'Do interventions that improve immunisation uptake also reduce social inequalities in uptake?' *British Medical Journal* 308: 1142–4.

Redmond, E., Rudd, A.G. and Martin, F.C. (1996) 'Older people in receipt of home help: a group with high levels of unmet health needs', *Health and Social Care in the Community* 4(6): 347–52.

Reuler, J.C. (1993) 'The American Experience', in K. Fisher and J. Collins (eds) *Homelessness, Health Care and Welfare Provision*, London: Routledge.

Richardson, D. (1994) 'Inclusion and exclusion: lesbians, HIV and AIDS', in L. Doyal, J. Naidod and T. Wilton (eds) *AIDS Setting a Feminist Agenda*, London: Taylor and Francis.

Richardson, S. and Pearson, M. (1995) 'Dignity and aspirations denied: unmet health and social care needs in an inner-city area', *Health and Social Care in the Community* 3(5): 279–87.

Rigge, M. (1993) *The Quality of Life of Long-wait Orthopaedic Patients Before and After Admission to Hospital*, London: College of Health.

—— (1994) 'Quality of life for long-wait orthopaedic patients before and after admission: a consumer audit', *Quality in Health Care* 3: 159–63.

Rivers, I. (1995) 'Mental health issues among young lesbians and gay men bullied in school', *Health and Social Care in the Community* 3(6): 380–3.

Road Haulage Association (1999) *Transport Policy*, London: http://www.rah.net/rha/policy_main.html

Roberts, H. (1985) *The Patient Patients: Women and their Doctors*, London: Pandora.

Roberts, H., Smith, S. and Bryce, C. (1993) 'Prevention is better ...', *Sociology of Health and Illness* 15(4): 447–63.

Roberts, H., Pearson, J.C.G., Madeley, R.J., Hanford, S. and Magowan, R. (1997) 'Unemployment and health: the quality of social support among residents in the Trent region of England', *Journal of Epidemiology and Community Health* 51: 41–5.

Roberts, I. (1997) 'Cause-specific social class mortality differentials for child injury and poisoning in England and Wales', *Journal of Epidemiology and Community Health* 51: 334–5.

Roberts, I. and Power, C. (1996) 'Does the decline in childhood injury mortality vary by social class? A comparison of class-specific mortality in 1981 and 1991', *British Medical Journal* 313: 784–6.

Rodberg, L. and Stevenson, G. (1977) 'The health care industry in advanced capitalism', *The Review of Radical Economics* 9(1): 104–15.

Rodgers, J. (1994) 'Primary health care provision for people with learning difficulties', *Health and Social Care in the Community* 2: 11–17.

Rosenfield, M. and Smillie, E. (1998) 'Group counselling by telephone', *British Journal of Counselling* 26(1): 11–19.

Rosenfield, M. And Urben, L. (1994) *Running a telephone cancer support group. Evaluation of a short term project*, London: Cancerlink.

Ross, F. and Tissier, J. (1997) 'The care management interface with general practice: a case study', *Health and Social Care in the Community* 5(3): 153–61.

Rothwell, P.M., McDowell, Z., Wong, C.K. and Dorman, P.J. (1997) 'Doctors and patients don't agree: cross-sectional study of patients' and doctors' perceptions and assessments of disability in multiple sclerosis', *British Medical Journal* 314: 1580–3.

Ruane, S. (1997) 'Public–private boundaries and the transformation of the NHS', *Critical Social Policy* 17(2): 53–78.

Rubin, G., Garvican, L. and Moss, S. (1998) 'Routine invitation of women aged 65–69 for breast cancer screening: results of first year of pilot study', *British Medical Journal* 317: 388–9.

Rudat, K. (1994) *Health and Lifestyles; Black and Minority Ethnic Groups in England*, London: Health Education Authority.

Russell, J. (1989) *South Glamorgan Care for the Elderly Hospital Discharge Service*, Cardiff: Cardiff University, School of Social and Administrative Studies.

Rumsey, N. and Harcourt, D. (1998) 'The care of women with breast cancer: research, policy and practice', in L. Doyal (ed.) *Women and Health Services*, Buckingham: Open University Press.

Salter, B. (1995) 'The private sector and the NHS: redefining the welfare state', *Policy and Politics* 23(1): 17–30.

Samaritans (1997a) *Statistics*, Slough: The Samaritans.

—— (1997b) *Behind the Mask: Men's Feelings and Suicide*, Slough: The Samaritans.

Saunders, C. (1996) 'Into the valley of the shadow of death', *British Medical Journal* 313: 1599–601.

Save the Children (1995) *You're On Your Own*, London: Save the Children.

Schurdell, S., Pendleton, E., Tate, L., Trice, R. and Steward, P. (1995) 'Providing continuity in a "firm" case management system', *Nursing Management* 26, November (11): 42–4.

Schwartz, J., Slater, D., Larson, T., Pierson, W. and Koenig, J. (1993) 'Particulate air pollution and hospital emergency room visits for asthma in Seattle', *American Review of Respiratory Disease* 147: 826–31.

Scott-Samuel, A., Birley, M. and Ardern, K. (1998) *The Merseyside Guidelines for Health Impact Assessment*, Liverpool: University of Liverpool, Liverpool Public Health Observatory.

Seale, C. and Cartwright, A. (1994) *The Year Before Death*, Aldershot: Avebury.

Seale, C. F. (1989) 'What happens in hospices: a review of research evidence', *Social Science and Medicine*, 28(6): 551–9.

Sedgwick-Jell, S. (1996) 'Local authorities servicing health: rediscovering an historic role', in P. Bywaters and E. McLeod (eds) *Working for Equality in Health*, London: Routledge.

Shakespeare, T. (1995) 'Back to the future? New genetics and disabled people', *Critical Social Policy* 44/45: 22–35.

Sharma, U. (1992) *Complementary Medicine Today*, London: Routledge.

Shaw, A. (1991) *Review of Health-based Social Work in Avon*, Bristol: Avon Social Services.

Sheldon, F. (1997) *Psychosocial Palliative Care*, Cheltenham: Stanley Thornes.

Sidell, M. (1995) *Health in Old Age*, Buckingham: Open University Press.

Simpson, R.G. (1996) 'Relationships between self-help health organizations and professional health care providers', *Health and Social Care in the Community* 4(6): 359–70.

Skilbeck, J., Mott, L., Smith, D., Page, H. and Clark, D. (1997) 'Nursing care for people dying from chronic obstructive airways disease', *International Journal of Palliative Nursing* 3(2): 100–06.

Sloper, P. (1996) 'Needs and responses of parents following the diagnosis of childhood cancer', *Child: Care, Health and Development* 22(3): 187–202.

Smaje, C. (1995) *Health, 'Race' and Ethnicity: Making Sense of the Evidence*, London: Kings Fund Institute.

Smaje, C. and Le Grand, J. (1997) 'Ethnicity, equity and the use of health services in the British NHS', *Social Science and Medicine* 45(3): 485–96.

Small, N. (1997) 'Palliative care and HIV', *Agenda* 10, February–April: 6–7.

Smith, J., Gilford, S. and O'Sullivan, A. (1998) *The Family Background of Young Homeless People*, London: Family Policy Studies Centre.

Smith, R. (1996) 'Gap between death rates of rich and poor widens', *British Medical Journal* 314: 9.

—— (1998) 'Renegotiating medicine's contract with patients', *British Medical Journal* 316: 1622–3.

Social Services Inspectorate (SSI) (1992a) *Social Services for Hospital Patients I: Working at the Interface*, London: SSI, Department of Health.

—— (1992b) *Social Services for Hospital Patients II: The Implications for Community Care*, London: SSI, Department of Health.

—— (1993) *Social Services for Hospital Patients III: Users and Carers Perspectives*, London: SSI, Department of Health.

—— (1995a) *Moving On*, report on the national inspection of social services department arrangements for the discharge of older people from hospital to residential or nursing home care, London: SSI, Department of Health.

—— (1995b) *Moving On: A Further Year*, report on the national inspection of social services department arrangements for the discharge of older people from hospital to residential or nursing home care, London: SSI, Department of Health.

—— (1998a) *Inspection of Community Care Services for Black and Ethnic Minority Older People*, London: Department of Health.

—— (1998b) *Report of a Second Inspection of Arrangements for Assessment and Delivery of Home Care Services*, London: Department of Health.

Socialist Health Association (1996) SHA/SERA joint report 'Health and the Environment' sets agenda for government', *Socialism and Health* 4, October: 3.

Soothill, K., Mackay, L. and Webb, C. (eds) (1995) *Interprofessional Relations in Health Care*, London: Edward Arnold.

Spackman, A. (1991) *The Health of Informal Carers*, Southampton: Southampton University, Institute for Health and Policy Studies.

Spencer, N. (1996) 'Reducing child health inequalities: insights and strategies for health workers', in P. Bywaters and E. McLeod (eds) *Working for Equality in Health*, London: Routledge.

Stacey, M. (1988) *The Sociology of Health and Healing*, London: Unwin Hyman.

Standing, K. (1997) 'Scrimping, saving and schooling: lone mothers and 'choice' in education', *Critical Social Policy* 17(2): 79–99.

Stewart, G. and Stewart, J. (1993) *Social Work and Housing*, Basingstoke: Macmillan.

Stonewall (1996a) *Join the Campaign for Civil Rights*, London: Stonewall.

—— (1996b) *Queerbashing – A National Survey on Homophobic Violence and Harassment: Summary*, London: Stonewall.

Sykes, N.P., Pearson, S.E. and Chell, S. (1992) 'Quality of care of the terminally ill: the carers' perspective', *Palliative Medicine* 6: 227–36.

Tanner, D. (1998) 'Empowerment and care management: swimming against the tide', *Health and Social Care in the Community* 6(6): 447–57.

Taylor, I. and Robertson, A. (1994) 'The health needs of gay men: a discussion of the literature and implications for nursing', *Journal of Advanced Nursing* 20: 560–6.

Tebbit, P. (1998) 'Looking to the future: a report from the National Hospice Council for Hospice and Specialist Palliative Care Services', paper presented to the Help the Hospices Annual National Conference in association with the NHCSPCS, London.

The Big Issue (1997), 17–23 March.

The Big Issue in the North (1997) Annual Report and Accounts, Manchester: The Big Issue in the North.

The Terrence Higgins Trust (1998) web site: http://www.tht.org.uk.

The Terrence Higgins Trust and the Centre for Medical Law and Ethics, Kings College, London (1994) *Living Will*, London: The Terrence Higgins Trust, Kings College.

Thornton, P. and Hams, T. (1996) *Local Agenda 21/Anti-Poverty and Regeneration: Relationships and Prospects*, London: Local Government Management Board.

Thorogood, N. (1989) 'Afro-Caribbean women's experience of the health service', *New Community* 15(3): 319–34.

Townsend, J., Dyer, S., Cooper, T., Meade, T., Piper, M. and Frank, A. (1992) 'Emergency hospital admissions and readmissions of patients aged over 75 years and the effects of a community-based discharge scheme', *Health Trends* 24(4): 136–9.

Townsend, J., Frank, A. O., Fermont, D., Dyer, S., Karran, O. and Walgrove, A. (1990) 'Terminal cancer care and patients' preference for place of death: a prospective study', *British Medical Journal* 301: 415–7.

Townsend, J., Piper, M., Frank, A.O., Dyer, S., North, W.R.S. and Meade, T.W. (1988) 'Reduction in hospital readmission – stay of elderly patients by a community-based discharge scheme: a randomised controlled trial', *British Medical Journal* 297: 544–7.

Townsend, P. (1995) 'Poverty: Home and Away', *Poverty* 91, Summer 95: 9–12.

Trades Union Congress (1999) *Out of Breath and Out of Work*, London: Trades Union Congress.

Treasure, T. (1998) 'Lessons from the Bristol case', *British Medical Journal* 316: 1685–6.

Tree, D. (1997) *Removing the Barriers. The Case for a New Deal for Social Services and Security*, London: Local Government Association.

Tritter, J. (1996) *Patient-centred cancer services? What patients say*, Oxford: The National Cancer Alliance.

Turner, B. S. (1995) *Medical Power and Social Knowledge*, London: Sage.

Veitch, D. (1995) *Prescribing Citizen's Advice. An Evaluation of the Work of the Citizen's Advice Bureau with Health and Social Services in Birmingham*, Birmingham: Citizen's Advice Bureau.

Venn, M.J., Darling, E., Dickens, C., Quine, L., Rutter, D.R. and Slevin, M.L. (1996) 'The experience and impact of contracting a cancer information service', *European Journal of Cancer Care* 5: 38–42.

Victor, C. (1991) *Health and Health Care in Later Life*, Buckingham: Open University Press.

Waddington, E. and Henwood, M. (1996) *Going Home: An Evaluation of British Red Cross Home from Hospital Schemes*, London: British Red Cross Society.

Wainwright, D. (1996) 'The political transformation of the health inequalities debate', *Critical Social Policy* 16(4): 67–82.

Warden, J. (1998) 'New UK hospital careplan for elderly', *British Medical Journal* 317: 1340.

Warren, L. (1997) 'Health and Leisure in Asian Communities', *Community Care* 29 May–4 June: 26.

Warwick, I. (1993) 'Exploring informal sector care: the need for assessed, evaluated and resourced support', in P. Aggleton, P. Davies and G. Hart (eds) *AIDS: Facing the Second Decade*, London: The Falmer Press.

Watney, S. (1996) 'The politics of AIDS treatment information activism: a partisan view', in P. Bywaters and E. McLeod (eds) *Working for Equality in Health*, London: Routledge.

Watt, D. (1996) 'All together now: why social deprivation matters to everyone', *British Medical Journal* 312: 1026–9.

Watters, C. (1996) 'Representations and realities: black people, community care and mental illness', in W.I.U. Ahmad and K. Atkin (eds) *'Race' and Community Care*, Buckingham: Open University Press.

Weaver, R. (1996) 'Localities and inequalities: locality management in the inner city', in P. Bywaters and E. McLeod (eds) *Working for Equality in Health*, London: Routledge.

Weich, S. and Lewis, G. (1998) 'Poverty, unemployment and common mental disorders: population-based cohort study', *British Medical Journal* 317: 115–19.

Wesson, J.S. (1997) 'Meeting the informational, psychosocial and emotional needs of each ICU patient and family', *Intensive and Critical Care Nursing* 13, April (2): 111–8.

White, C. (1998) 'Patients at risk as staff crisis grows', *Nursing Times* 94(42): 5.

Whitehead, M. (1987) *The Health Divide*, London: Harmondsworth, Penguin.

Whiteley, P. (1997) 'Elderly miss out on benefits', *Community Care* 10–16 April: 6.

Whitfield, D. (1997) 'Why the private finance initiative poses the biggest threat to the NHS', *Socialism and Health* June: 4–5.

Wilkinson, R. (1992) 'Income distribution and life expectancy', *British Medical Journal* 304: 165–8.

—— (1994a) 'Divided We Fall', *British Medical Journal* 308: 1113–14.

—— (1994b) *Unfair Shares*, Ilford: Barnardos.

—— (1996a) *Unhealthy Societies*, London: Routledge.

—— (1996b) 'How can secular improvements in life expectancy be explained?' in D. Blane, E. Brunner and R. Wilkinson (eds) *Health and Social Organisation*, London and New York: Routledge.

Williams, F. (1992) 'Women with learning difficulties are women too', in M. Langan and L. Day (eds) *Women, Oppression and Social Work*, London: Routledge.

Williams, J. and Corcoran, G. (1996) *Palliative Care Prescribing*, Liverpool: North West Drug Information Service and Aintree Hospitals NHS Trust.

Williams, J.M., Currie, C.E., Wright, P., Elton, R.A. and Beattie, T.F. (1996) 'Socioeconomic status and adolescent injuries', *Social Science and Medicine* 44(12): 1881–91.

Williams, S. (1993) *Chronic Respiratory Illness*, London: Routledge.

Williams, S.J. and Calnan, M. (eds) (1996) *Modern Medicine*, London: UCL Press.

Wilson, I.M., Bunting, J.S., Curnow, R.N., Knock, J. (1995) 'The need for in-patient palliative care facilities for non-cancer patients in the Thames Valley', *Palliative Medicine* 9: 13–18.

Wilton, T. (1998) 'Gender, sexuality and healthcare: improving services' in L. Doyal (ed.) *Women and Health Services*, Buckingham: Open University Press.

Wistow, G. and Lewis, H. (1996) *Preventative Services for Older People: Current Approaches and Future Opportunities*, Kidlington, Oxon: Anchor Trust.

Woodrofe, C., Glickman, M., Barker, M. and Power, C. (1993) *Children, Teenagers and Health: The Key Data*, Buckingham: Open University Press.

WPCGPC (1997) *Changing Gear – Guidelines for Managing the Last Days of Life in Adults*, London: National Council for Hospice and Specialist Palliative Care Services.

—— (1998) *Guidelines for Managing Cancer Pain in Adults*, second edition, London: National Council for Hospice and Specialist Palliative Care Services.

World Health Organisation (1997) *The Jakarta Declaration on Health Promotion into the 21st Century*, http://www.ens.gu.edu.au/eberhard/jakdec.htm.

Worrall, A., Rea, J.N. and Ben-Shlomo, Y. (1997) 'Counting the cost of social disadvantage in primary care: retrospective analysis of patient data', *British Medical Journal* 314: 38–42.

Wyke, S., Hunt, K. and Ford, G. (1998) 'Gender differences in consulting a general practitioner for common symptoms of minor illness', *Social Science and Medicine* 46(7): 901–6.

Yates, J. (1995) *Private Eye, Heart and Hip*, London: Churchill Livingstone.

Young, M. and Cullen, L. (1996) *A Good Death*, London: Routledge.

Index

T - #0167 - 071024 - C0 - 216/138/13 - PB - 9780415164900 - Gloss Lamination